Inflammatory Diseases of the Orbit

Springer

Berlin
Heidelberg
New York
Barcelona
Hong Kong
London
Milan
Paris
Singapore
Tokyo

Renate Unsöld · Gabriele Greeven

Inflammatory Diseases of the Orbit

Clinical Features · Radiology
Differential Diagnosis

With a Foreword by A. R. Margulis

Translated by S. Schneider

With 495 Partly Colored Illustrations

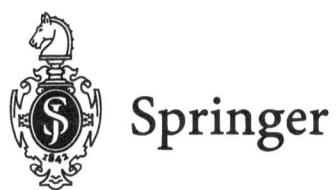

Springer

Renate Unsöld, MD
Professor of Ophthalmology
Heinrich Heine University
Blumenstraße 28, D-40212 Düsseldorf
Germany

Gabriele Greeven, MD
Clinic of Diagnostic Radiology
St. Elisabeth-Hospital
Friedrich-Ebert-Straße 56, D-56564 Neuwied
Germany

Translator
Stephany Schneider, MD
Im Schlangenkamp 9, D-44623 Herne
Germany

ISBN-13: 978-3-642-64042-1   e-ISBN-13: 978-3-642-59597-4
DOI: 10.1007/978-3-642-59597-4

Translated from the German edition R. Unsöld/G. Greeven, *Entzündliche Orbitaerkrankungen*,
© Springer-Verlag Berlin Heidelberg 1997

Library of Congress Cataloging-in-Publication Data

Unsöld, R. (Renate), 1946– . [Entzündliche Orbitaerkrankungen. English]. Inflammatory diseases of
the orbit : clinical features, radiology, differential diagnosis / Renate Unsöld and Gabriele Greeven. p. cm.
Includes bibliographical references and index.   1. Eye-
sockets – Inflammation. I. Greeven, Gabriele. II. Title. [DNLM: 1. Orbital Diseases – diagnosis. 2. Diagnosis. Differential. 3. Inflammation – diagnosis. 4. Tomography, X-Ray Computed. WW 202 U59e
1999a]. RE711.U5513 1999. 617.7'8 – dc21. DNLM/DLC. for Library of Congress. 99-41443

© Springer-Verlag Berlin Heidelberg 2000

Softcover reprint of the hardcover 1st edition 2000

Product liability: The publishers cannot guarantee the accuracy of any information about dosage and
application contained in this book. In every individual case the user must check such information by con-
sulting the relevant literature.

Cover design: Erich Kirchner, Heidelberg
Typesetting: Fotosatz-Service Köhler GmbH, 97084 Würzburg
Computer to film and binding: Universitätsdruckerei Stürtz AG, 97080 Würzburg

SPIN: 10693978   21/3135 – 5 4 3 2 1 0 – Printed on acid-free paper

Dedicated to our teachers and friends

Jack DeGroot
Alexander R. Margulis
and Thomas H. Newton

We thank the
„Verein zur Förderung der Augenheilkunde in Düsseldorf e.V."
and the chairmen for their generous support
with the color reproduction.

Foreword

This concise, beautifully illustrated book translated from a highly success-
ful edition in German is a pleasure to read. The well-organized text is
correlated with high-quality color photographs of patients, as well as CT
sections through the orbits with reformatted images when this approach
clarifies the case illustration. The few pictures of pathologic specimens
and anatomic cross-sections further enhance the didactic value of the
monograph.

The book is organized by presenting the history, clinical findings (illustrated in color), and CT sections through the orbit of patients afflicted
with the disease that is described. This is followed by the diagnosis and a
concise discussion of the course and treatment, emphasizing the pathologic
features of the condition. The presentation of each of the multiple inflammatory diseases affecting the orbit or eye are followed by many actual case
presentations illustrating the various aspects of the specific disease.

The book begins with an introduction and review of the general aspects
of diagnosis of orbital diseases, again well illustrated. The main conditions
dealt with in detail in subsequent chapters are: Graves' disease; inflammatory orbital pseudotumor; inflammatory diseases of the lacrimal gland;
orbital inflammations associated with those of the paranasal sinuses. The
differential diagnosis is given in each case. The last three chapters display
the teaching originality of the authors: In Chap. 7 cases are selected solely
for the presentation of important teaching points. While Chap. 8 presents
similar CT findings in patients suffering from different diseases, Chap. 9
shows CT images of 13 patients with findings sufficiently characteristic to
strongly suggest a specific diagnosis.

The whole approach of this book is highly original. The meticulous attention to the clinical features of inflammatory diseases of the orbit, with
excellent illustrations, makes reading it and learning from it fun.

Alexander R. Margulis

Contents

1 Introduction

Inflammations of orbital tissues represent the majority of orbital diseases. It is frequently difficult to differentiate them from each other as well as from other pathological processes, particularly from neoplasms. It is almost impossible to establish a safe diagnosis on the basis of clinical findings alone.

Thin-section computed tomography (CT) is still the examination method of choice in the differentiation of pathological processes of the viscerocranial region and the skull base. In some cases ultrasound and magnetic resonance imaging (MRI) may add useful differential diagnostic information. In most cases diagnosis can be established with safety on the basis of a careful history, clinical signs and symptoms, and the CT appearance.

In special clinical situations, for instance in soft-tissue masses and dense infiltrations, CT shows the optimal route to surgical biopsy.

We set out to give a concise, systematic survey of the clinical signs and symptoms and the characteristic CT patterns of different inflammatory disease entities. The most important clinical and CT criteria for differential diagnosis are defined and evaluated. To give the reader the opportunity to develop a more profound understanding of differential diagnostic criteria, selected case reports of clinically and histologically confirmed cases are presented. We decided not to group the case reports in order to minimize any bias that might arise from the fact that a case report appears in a certain chapter.

Relevant reviews and original articles pertinent to the differential diagnosis of inflammatory orbital lesions are listed at the end of the book, we deliberately kept this section short.

The case reports, selected from more than 4000 cases treated during the past 15 years, approximately 1000 of which are documented in teaching files, were chosen for didactic reasons.

Introduction

2 General Aspects of the Diagnosis of Inflammatory Diseases of the Orbit

Some disease entities involving the orbit can be diagnosed quite safely on the basis of the clinical findings, for instance typical Graves' disease (Case 1). Frequently, however, anatomical and clinical variations disguise typical features (Cases 28, 30, 31, 33, 34). On the other hand, it is remarkable how often almost identical clinical aspects may be seen in disease entities of entirely different etiology. Impressive examples illustrating this phenomenon include subperiosteal abscesses, malignant tumors, and nonspecific inflammatory processes, which require completely different therapeutic measures (Cases 3–26). In addition there is a surprising diversity of clinical aspects of one and the same disorder, for instance in Graves' disease (Cases 27–34).

Similar phenomena occur in the evaluation of CT and MR images. Many disease entities can quite safely be diagnosed on the basis of CT and MRI. Others require detailed knowledge of the clinical symptomatology. Enlargement of extraocular muscles or diffuse orbital infiltration, for example, may be caused by lesions of quite different etiology (cf. p. 173–180, Plates 15, 16). It is therefore important to consider not only the clinical appearance but also to take a comprehensive history, including surgery and trauma, and immunological disorders of the patient and his or her direct relatives.

All information regarding history and clinical findings should be shared with the radiologist in order to give him the chance to choose the examination technique that makes the best use of the diagnostic capacity of the modality concerned. This is obvious, for instance, in the diagnosis of venous malformations, many of which can be detected only when the patient's head is positioned downwards (Case 106). If the diagnosis cannot be established with safety on the basis of clinical and radiological findings, ENT and internal medical examinations, biopsy may prove necessary.

In unilateral space-occupying lesions of the lacrimal gland, however, one should be extremely cautious: if a primary epithelial neoplasm of the lacrimal gland cannot be ruled out, primary en-bloc resection should be performed. Particularly in benign mixed tumors of the lacrimal gland, the rate of recurrence, malignancy, and mortality increases considerably after biopsy or partial resection. In these cases primary en-bloc resection including the adjacent bone is mandatory.

History Taking

Because inflammatory orbital disease and its differential diagnosis comprises such a broad spectrum of etiologically different disease entities, detailed history taking, incorporating family history as well as systemic inflammatory, autoimmune and malignant disease, is essential. It is important also to ask about previous trauma and surgery. Explicit exploration frequently reveals findings highly relevant for the interpretation of CT or MR images. The answers may provide clues to the explanation of bone defects, intramuscular hematoma, intraorbital emphysema, systemic granulomatous inflammation, or foreign body reactions. It is important not to miss trauma and surgery that took place long ago, since complications may emerge many years later. The development of a mucocele, for example, or the shrinking of a paranasal sinus may be delayed side effects of paranasal-sinus surgery. Posttraumatic arteriovenous cavernous sinus fistulas may also evolve after a considerable time. When interviewing children, one should bear in mind that they might be afraid to mention wounds or foreign body injuries brought about by forbidden activities.

There is, on the other hand, the risk of attributing serious pathological processes to minor trauma. Such mistakes impede adequate diagnostic and therapeutic measures. The resulting delay is particularly harmful for patients with malignant neoplasms such as rhabdomyosarcomas, neuroblastomas, or leukemic infiltrations, in which immediate intervention is needed.

Many inflammatory processes affecting the orbit develop from pathological reactions of the immune system, e.g. Graves' disease, certain kinds of the inflammatory pseudotumor or intraorbital tumors as seen in association with panarteritis nodosa or Wegener's granulomatosis. Since most systemic inflammatory diseases are to some extent inherited defects of the immune system, it is important to take a thorough and comprehensive family history. It is by no means rare for a patient to develop more than one autoimmune disease during his or her life. Awareness of any previous autoimmune disease facilitates the diagnosis of the present disease.

Inquiries should also be made with regard to previous as well as on going infections of the respiratory tract and any antibiotic or anti-inflammatory medication taken. Complications of bacterial sinusitis can then be recognized as such even if they are, owing to drug therapy, present in an atypical or mitigated form. Since the orbit is quite often the first site of manifestation of metastases or of leukemic infiltrations, a detailed history of internal medical disease and pathological laboratory findings is important.

If a patient presents with a habitus suggestive of acromegaly, one should bear in mind that diffuse extraocular muscle enlargement may be associated with an adenoma of the pituitary gland even in the absence of any thyroid disorder (Case 45). The pathogenetic mechanisms responsible for this phenomenon remain to be investigated.

Optimal Use of Imaging Techniques

Many incorrect and delayed diagnoses and their frequently serious sequelae could have been avoided had the most suitable imaging technique been chosen.

Lesions within the anterior two-thirds of the orbit, such as cavernous hemangiomas, cavernous sinus fistulas with their characteristic flow reversal, and enlargement of the extraocular muscles can be diagnosed with a high degree of certainty by standardized sonography. Lesions within the posterior third of the orbit and of the orbital bones, however, are for technical reasons frequently missed. To rely on ultrasonographic findings alone invariably leads to misinterpretations. This is particularly true for secondary changes of orbital tissues, due to lesions of the paranasal sinuses or other neighboring compartments, as in meningiomas of the sphenoid bone, malignomas, or necrotizing granulomas of the paranasal sinuses.

Many inflammatory diseases of the orbit and their differential diagnoses can be identified only

by using thin-section CT and computer reformating. Since most orbital structures and lesions differ considerably in density related to the hypodense surrounding orbital fat, the majority of pathologic processes confined to the orbit can be detected without the use of contrast media. Delineation of lesions originating within, or extending into, the intracranial space requires contrast enhancement. Some orbital venous malformations can only be visualized by positioning the patient's head downwards (Case 106).

Many inflammatory lesions of the orbit are accompanied by hyperostosis or erosion of the adjacent bone. Calcifications such as phleboliths within venous malformations, calcium deposits in sclerosing inflammations, or dense foreign bodies within foreign body granulomas can generally not be reliably visualized by MRI alone. This applies particularly to thick-section MRI, which does not allow clear delineation of pneumatized paranasal sinuses, bone, and vessels.

In our experience, thin-section CT, using an optimal plane of section and computer reformating, remains the examination technique of choice for primary evaluation of lesions of the orbit and skull base. MRI and ultrasound may add valuable information in particular cases. In general, neither CT nor MRI should be used for screening. The appropriate examination technique has to be carefully determined in each individual case.

The optimal plane of section for the radiological examination of the orbit is obtained at a negative angulation of approximately 20° to the orbitomeatal baseline or parallel to the McGregor line. These planes of section ensure optimal visualization of the optic canal and structures of the orbital apex. This is particularly important for diagnosing lesions extending from the orbit, via the superior orbital fissure or the optic canal, into the intracranial space, and vice versa, and for determining the topographic relationship of the optic nerve and the internal carotid artery within the intracranial end of the optic canal.

Interdisciplinary Cooperation

In many cases correct interpretation of radiological findings depends on detailed knowledge of the clinical situation. Diagnostic safety depends on the close cooperation of clinicians and radiologists. The closer the cooperation, the higher the chance of choosing the optimal examination technique with regard to the patient's particular problem and the higher the diagnostic safety. Close interdisciplinary cooperation reduces the number of false-negative results and diagnostic errors, thus saving the costs of unnecessary additional examinations.

Many inflammatory diseases of the orbit are, like their differential diagnoses, associated with systemic inflammatory or malignant disease. Close cooperation among clinicians, surgeons, and radiologists is particularly necessary in order to correctly interpret postoperative radiographic findings and to evaluate the effectiveness of various therapeutic measures.

Particularly in orbital complications of malignant neoplasms and chronic systemic diseases, the patient's life expectancy and quality of life depend on the effectiveness of interdisciplinary collaboration.

Characteristic Clinical Aspects of Inflammatory Orbital Diseases that Allow Diagnosis with a High Degree of Certainty

Plate 1

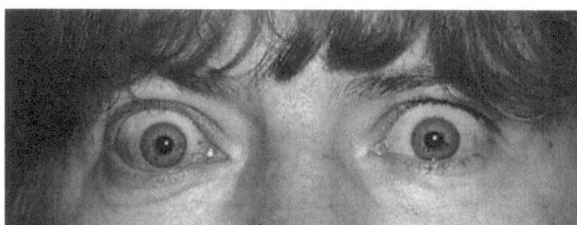

1

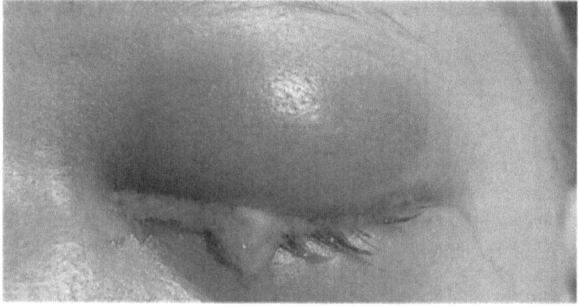

2

Diagnosis 1: Typical appearance of a patient with Graves' disease. Bilateral proptosis, lid retraction and periorbital swelling.

Diagnosis 2: Orbital cellulitis with purulent discharge.

Similar Aspects in Etiologically Different Diseases

Plate 2

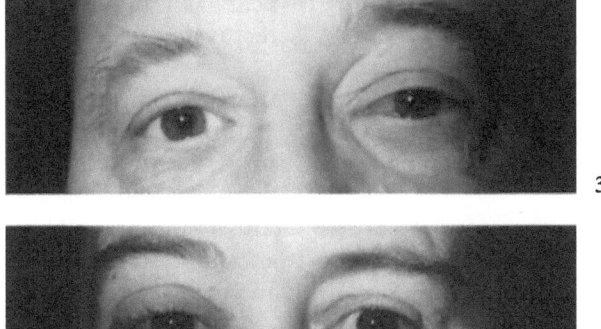

3

4

Both patients exhibit unilateral periorbital swelling
and hyperemia as well as proptosis and chemosis.

J.M., 49-year-old man

History and Clinical Findings

Endonasal surgery on the maxillary sinus and the ethmoidal air cells 1 year ago. Postoperatively, diplopia and pain. A space-occupying lesion in the region of the left medial rectus muscle was visualized by CT and MRI.

Medial orbitotomy for progressive visual loss 9 months later.

Exploratory surgery. Histopathology: pathological changes consistent with inflammatory orbital pseudotumor.

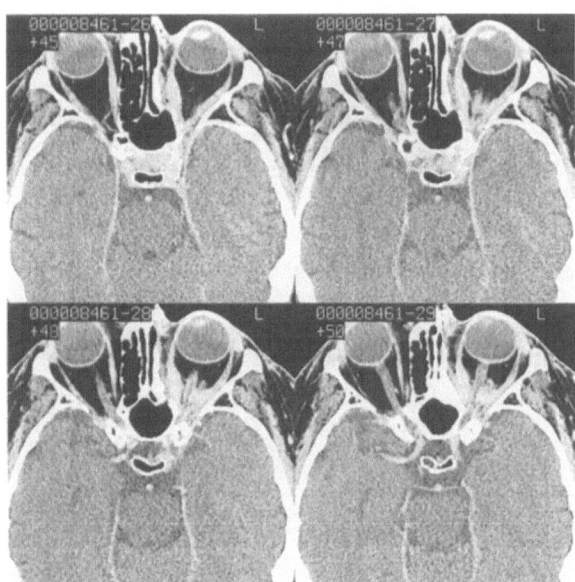

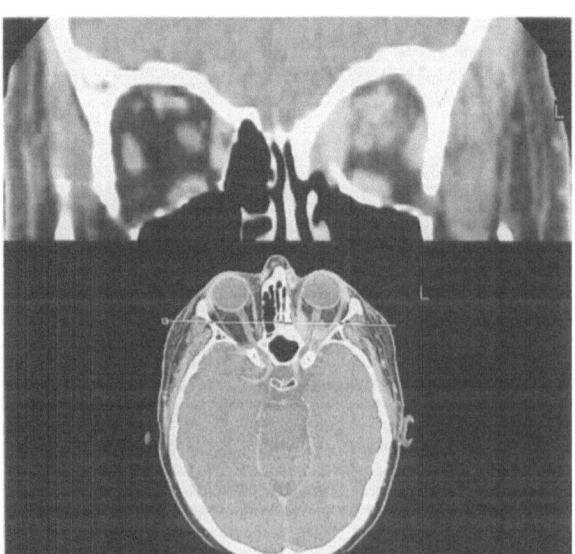

3.1

3.2

Steroid treatment. After dose reduction, recurrence of pain, restriction of ocular motility, and periorbital swelling.

CT (3.1 and 3.2)

State after radical surgery on the left ethmoidal air cells and medial orbitotomy. The medial orbital wall and parts of the orbital roof and the orbital floor have been removed. The resulting cavities are to some extent filled with soft-tissue masses extending into the orbital apex. The optic nerve appears as a hypodense band. The adjacent medial rectus muscle is enlarged and displaced medially.

Diagnosis

State after medial orbitotomy and after radical surgery on the left ethmoidal air cells. Extended bone defects in the medial orbital wall with large soft-tissue areas adjacent to the medial orbital wall and the orbital apex. Spindle-shaped enlargement and displacement of the medial rectus muscle.

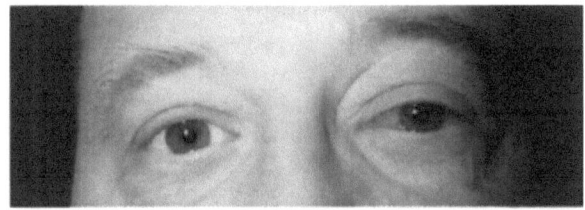

3.3

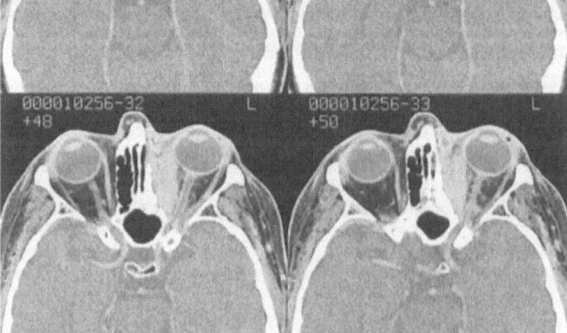

3.4

CT (3.4)

Eight months later. Increase in size of the soft-tissue masses with displacement of the medial rectus muscle.

Diagnosis
Recurrence of the reactive granulomatous inflammation.

Meanwhile, ocular muscle surgery had been performed in order to remove "scar tissue" around the medial rectus muscle. There was no improvement of diplopia. Clinical improvement after treatment with steroids for 3 months.

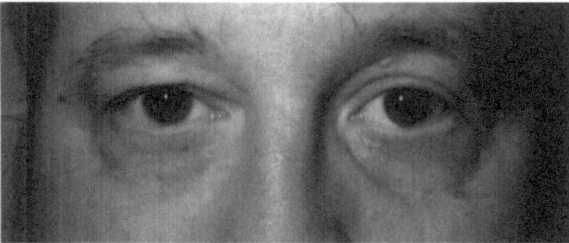

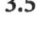
3.5

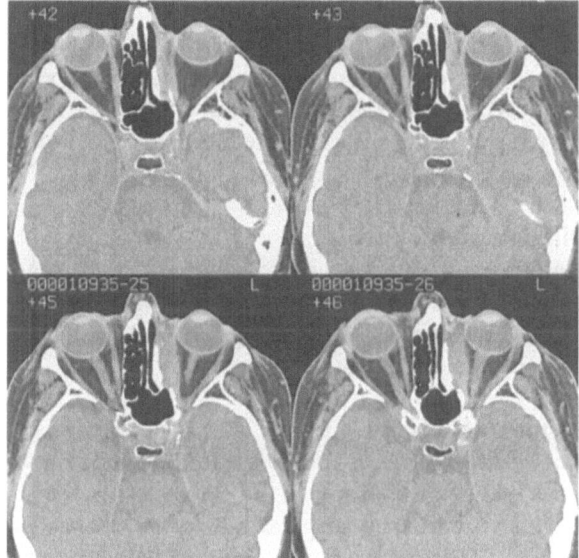
3.6

CT (3.6)
One year later. The cavity in the region of the left ethmoidal air cells is completely filled with homogeneous soft-tissue masses, within which the medial rectus muscle can hardly be identified. By comparison with the previous CT scans, overall shrinkage of soft-tissue masses.

Diagnosis
Scar formation within the post-surgical cavity.

Histopathology
Granulomatous inflammatory reaction. Wegener's granulomatosis was excluded.

K. K., 54-year-old woman

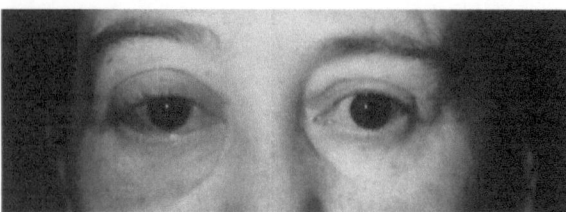

4.1

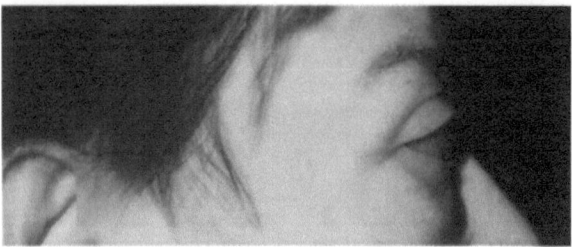

4.2

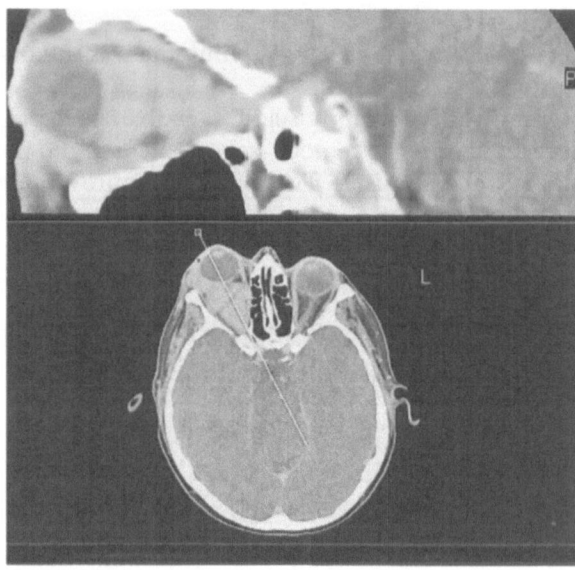

4.4

History and Clinical Findings
Protrusion of the right globe during the past 9 years. Considerable increase in proptosis the past 6 months.

Sensation of pressure behind the eye. Generalized restriction of ocular motility, and double vision in extreme right gaze. No visual loss. Lid swelling.

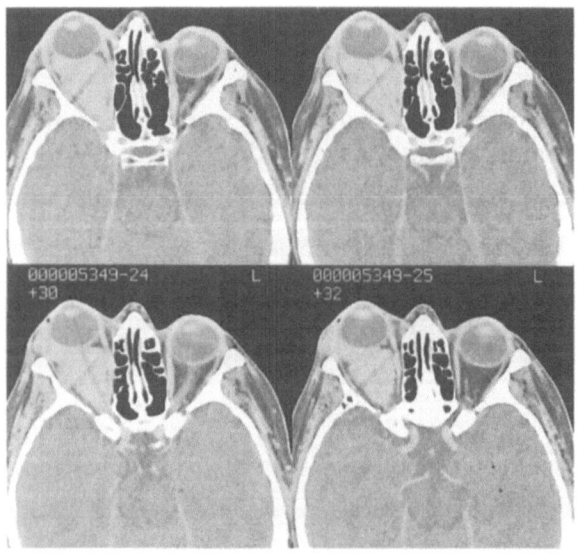

4.3

CT (4.3 and 4.4)
Large, well-defined, polycyclic, space-occupying lesion within the right intraconal space. The optic nerve appears as a hypodense band. Proptosis and impression of the posterior wall of the globe.

Differential Diagnosis
Meningioma of the optic nerve sheath, slowly growing lymphoma, inflammatory orbital pseudotumor, or metastasis of a malignant neoplasm.

A surgical biopsy is necessary.

Histopathology
Low-grade non-Hodgkin lymphoma (biopsy proven). Radiation therapy.

One month later, surgical biopsy of the gastric mucosa. Histopathological diagnosis: suspected MALT lymphoma. Seven months later, gastrectomy. Histopathological diagnosis: MALT lymphoma. Chemotherapy.

(Continued on p. 11)

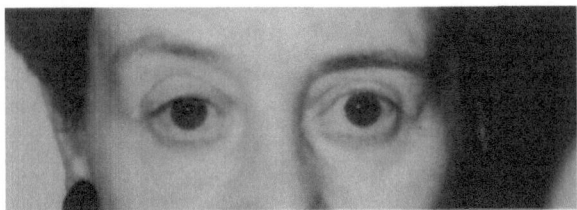

4.5

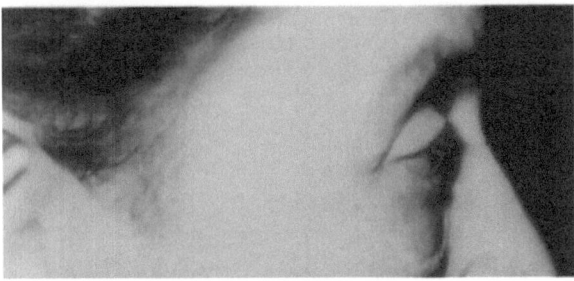

4.6

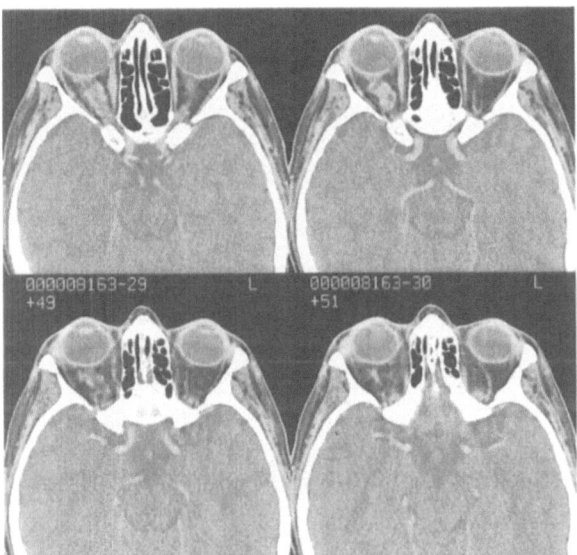

4.7

CT (4.7 and 4.8)
One year later. Areas of increased density surrounding the optic nerve, which appears as a hypodense band. Remission of proptosis.

Diagnosis
After radiation and chemotherapy remission of the biopsy-proven lymphoma.

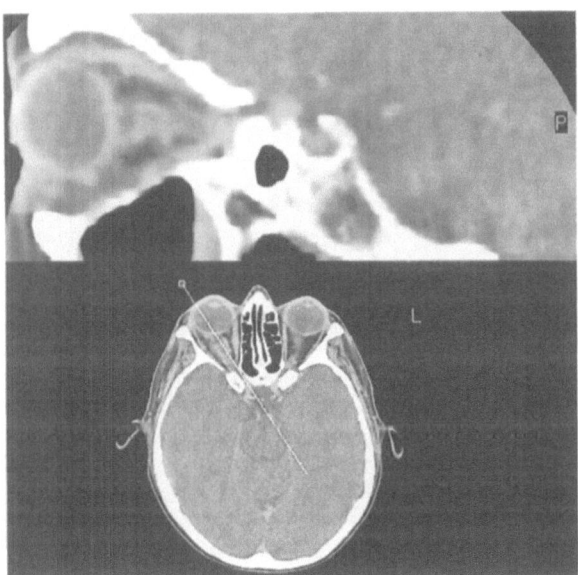

4.8

Plate 3

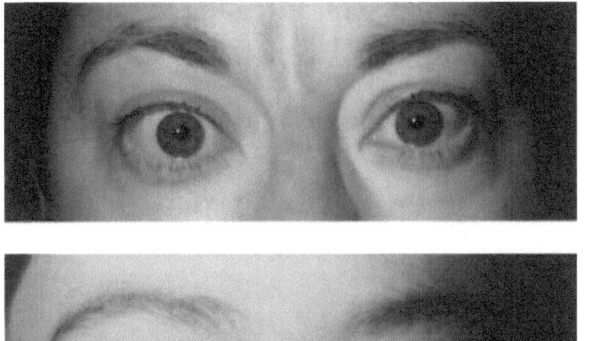

5

6

The palpebral fissures of both patients appear widened with lid retraction above the limbus.

W. B., 44-year-old woman

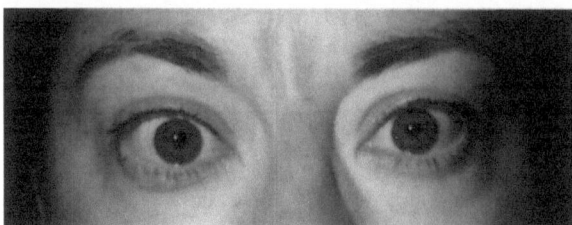

5.1

History and Clinical Findings
Proptosis, more prominent in the right eye.

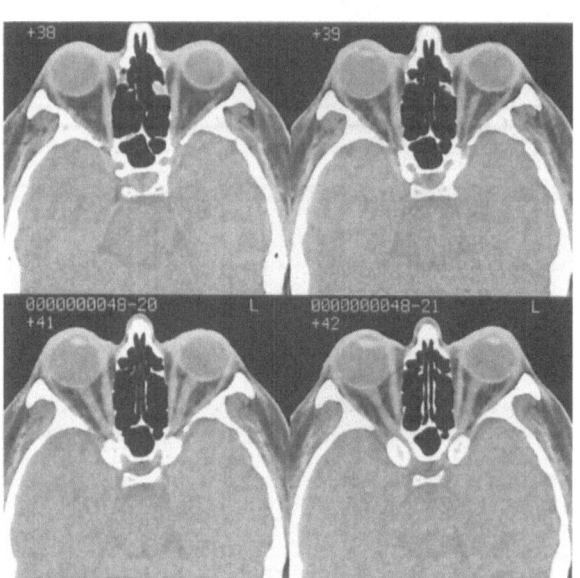

5.2

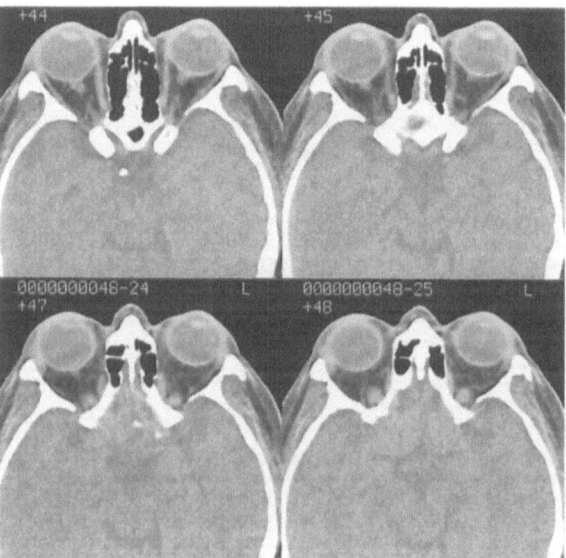

5.3

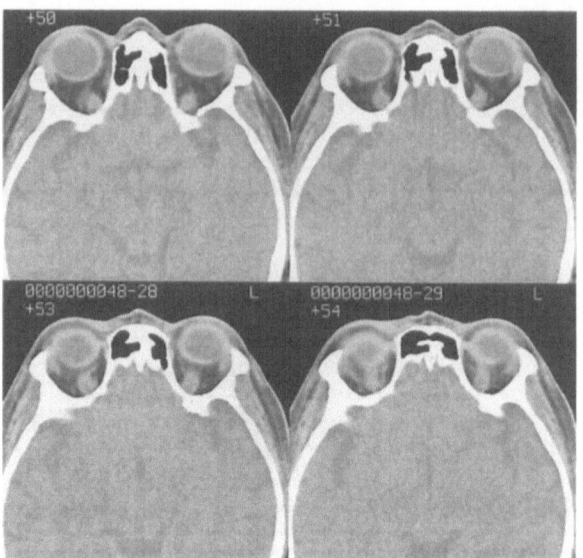

5.4

CT
Small bony orbits

Comment
Suspicion of Graves' disease is not confirmed by the CT findings. "Large eyes" since childhood.

P. G., 31-year-old woman

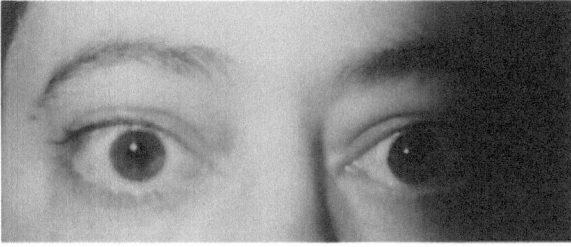

6.1

History and Clinical Findings

Hyperthyroidism and Graves' ophthalmopathy diagnosed 12 months ago. Initially antithyroid medication, near-total thyroidectomy 7 months ago. Steroid treatment was ineffective.

Bilateral proptosis, lid retraction, and restriction of upward gaze.

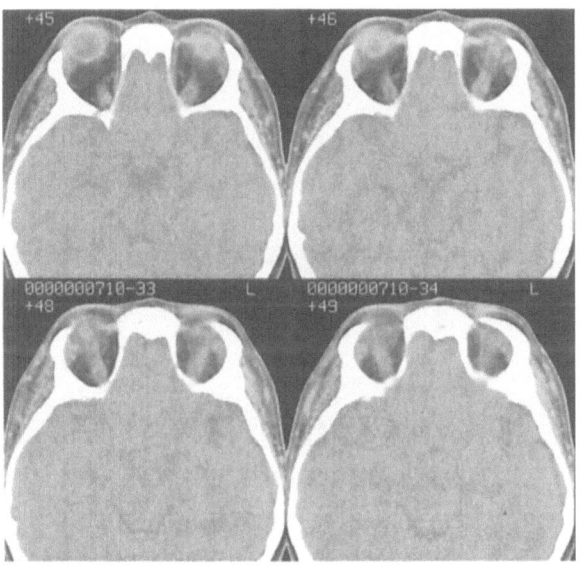

6.2

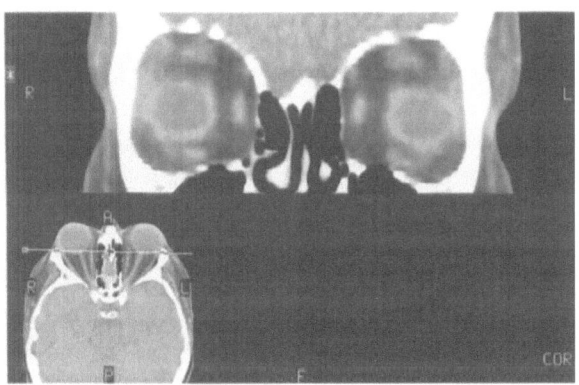

6.3

CT

Bilaterally, slight enlargement of the lacrimal gland and of the upper muscle complex. Increase in the volume of orbital fat.

Diagnosis

Graves' disease, predominantly dacryoadenitic form.

Plate 4

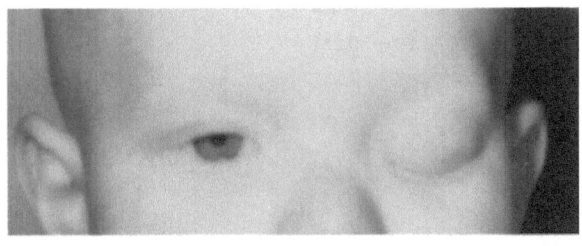

7

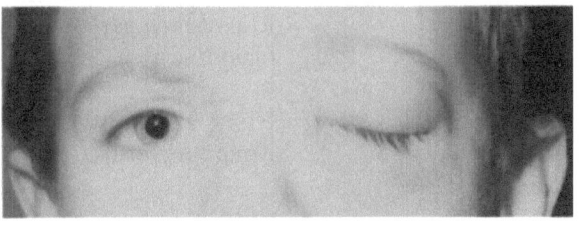

8

Both patients exhibit unilateral proptosis, swelling
of the left lid, and complete ptosis.

H. A., 4-month-old girl

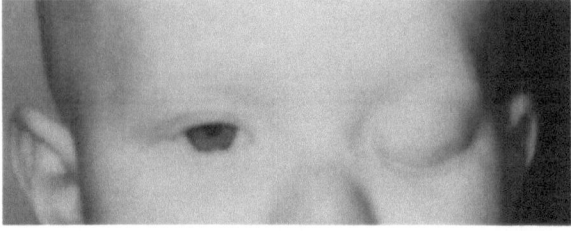

7.1

History and Clinical Findings
Increasing ptosis of the left lid for the past 2 months. Frequent crying. Normal EEG.

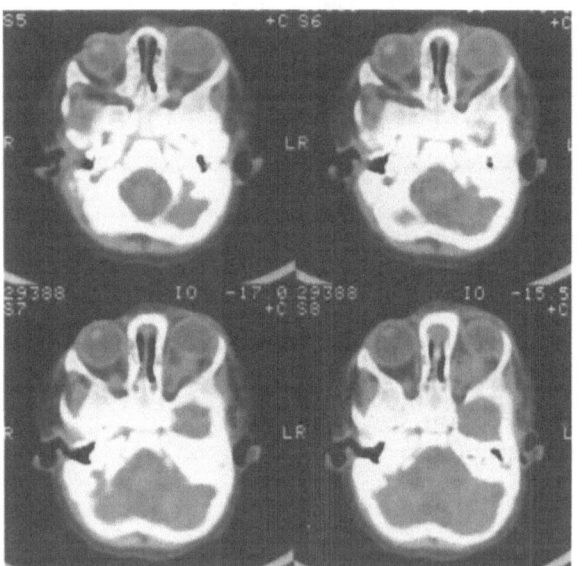

7.2

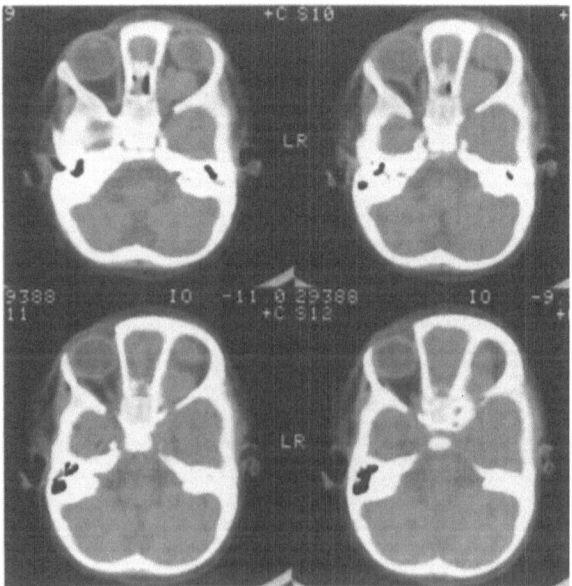

7.3

CT
Large, polycyclic, solid, space-occupying lesion within the left intraconal space.

Differential Diagnosis
Rhabdomyosarcoma or metastasis of a neuroblastoma.

Histopathology
Rhabdomyosarcoma.

Clinical Course
Chemotherapy, followed by complete remission.

Comment
The main differential diagnoses of intraconal space-occupying lesions in babies and small children are neuroblastoma and rhabdomyosarcoma.

The absence of bone destruction and of lesions in the paranasal sinuses, points to a diagnosis other than histiocytosis X or osteomyelitis.

B. O., 4-year-old boy

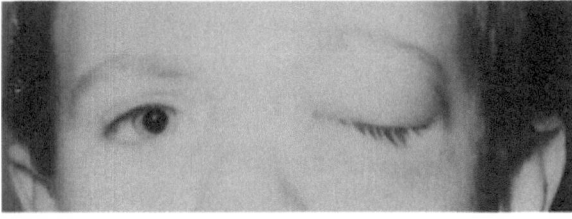

8.1

History and Clinical Findings
Rhinitis, "stuffy nose", and fever up to 101.8°F (38.8°C) for 2 weeks. Presently considerable periorbital swelling on the left side.

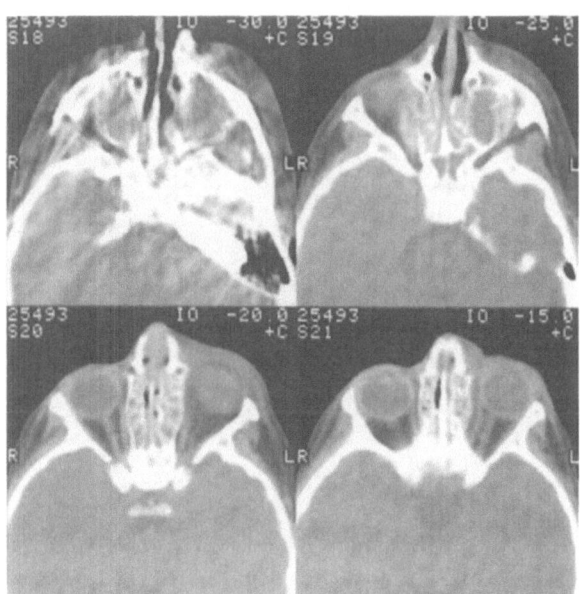

8.2

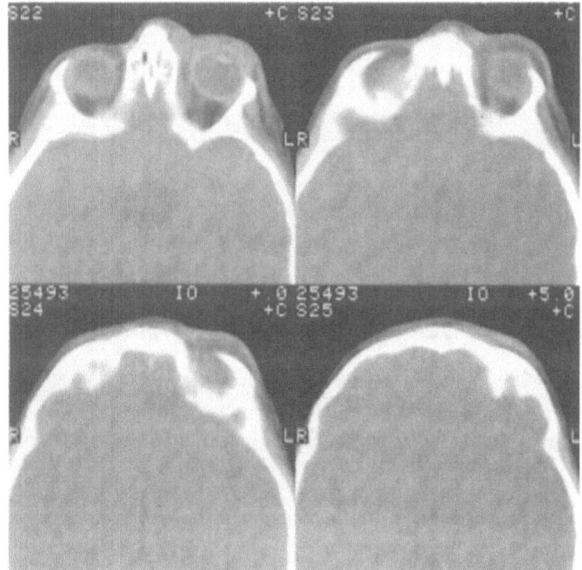

8.3

CT
Complete opacification of both maxillary sinuses and ethmoidal air cells. Soft-tissue swelling around the orbit. Well-defined area of increased density within the medial extraconal space. The adjacent medial rectus muscle is displaced laterally.

Diagnosis
Pansinusitis with periorbital cellulitis and a subperiosteal abscess.

Clinical Course
Complete remission after systemic antibiotic treatment.

Plate 5

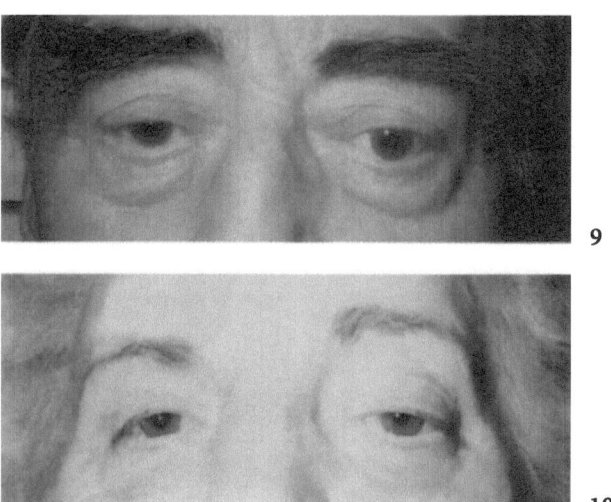

9

10

Both patients exhibit unilateral proptosis.

B. F., 77-year-old man

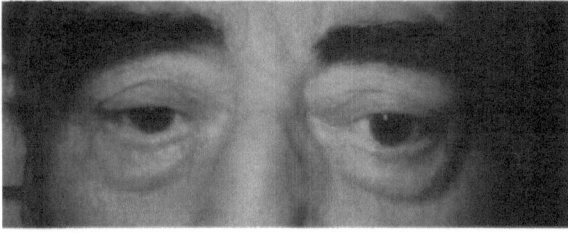

9.1

History and Clinical Findings

Hyperthyroidism diagnosed 6 years ago. Antithyroid medication.

Two years ago, normal thyroid function. For the past month increasing proptosis of the left eye, chemosis, hyperlacrimation, and double vision. Presently euthyroid.

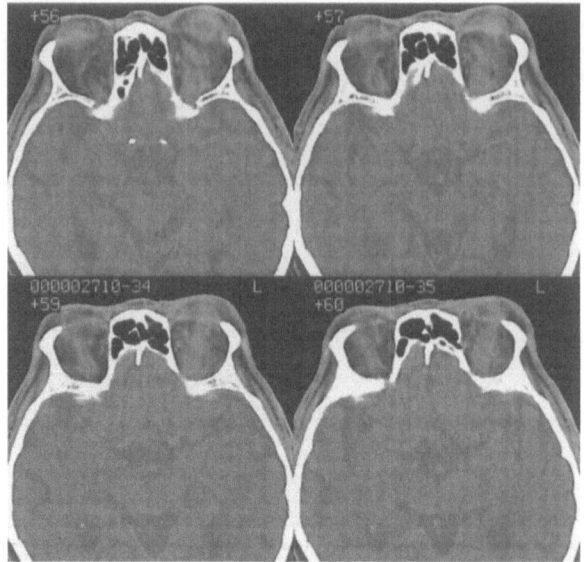

9.4

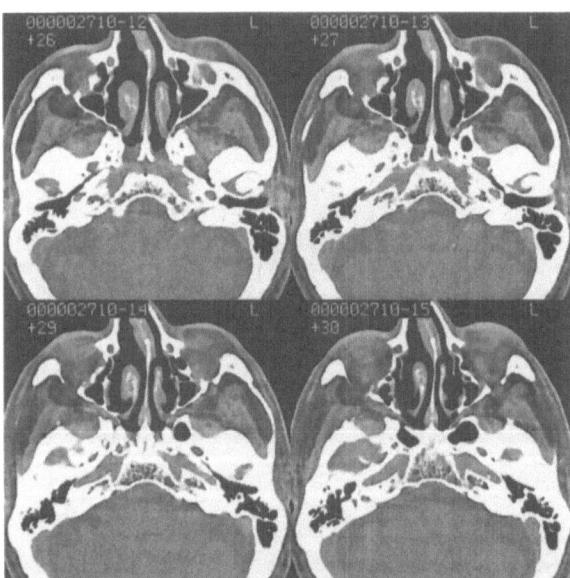

9.2

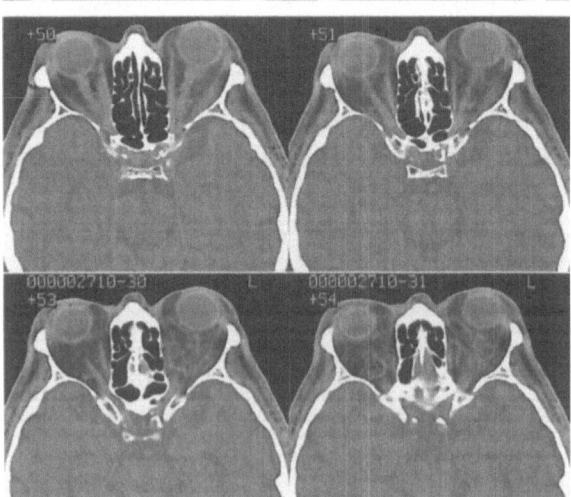

9.3

9.5

CT

Considerable enlargement of extraocular muscles. Dilatation of orbital veins. Asymmetrical proptosis, more pronounced on the left side. Erosion of the right orbital floor with herniation of orbital fat and spontaneous decompression.

Diagnosis

Polymyositic form of Graves' disease.

Comment

Due to spontaneous decompression, proptosis is much less pronounced on the right side.

W. C., 67-year-old woman

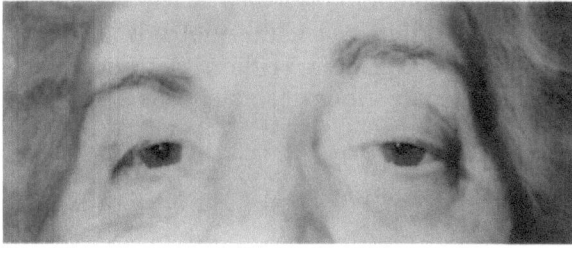

10.1

History and Clinical Findings
Increasing proptosis for many years, documented by photographs.

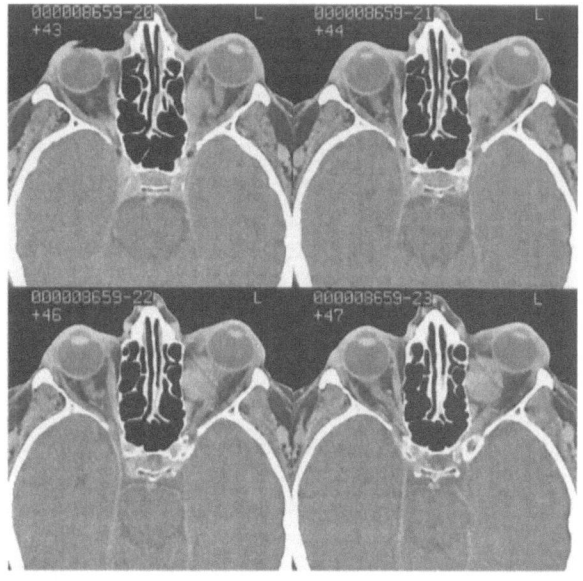

10.2

10.3

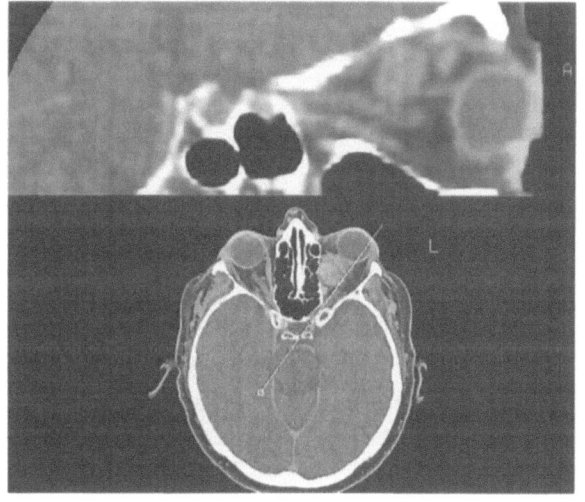

10.4

(Continued on p. 24)

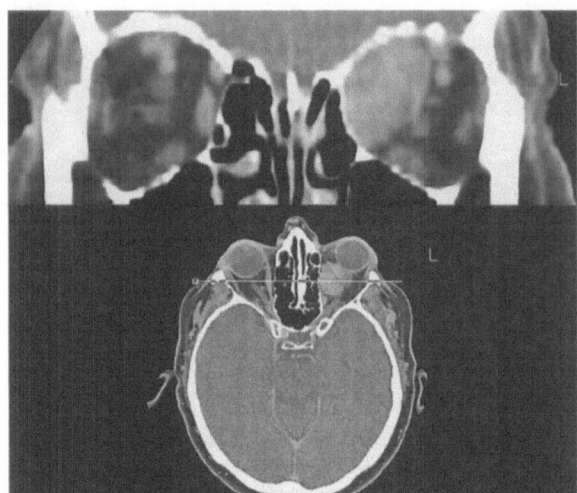

10.5

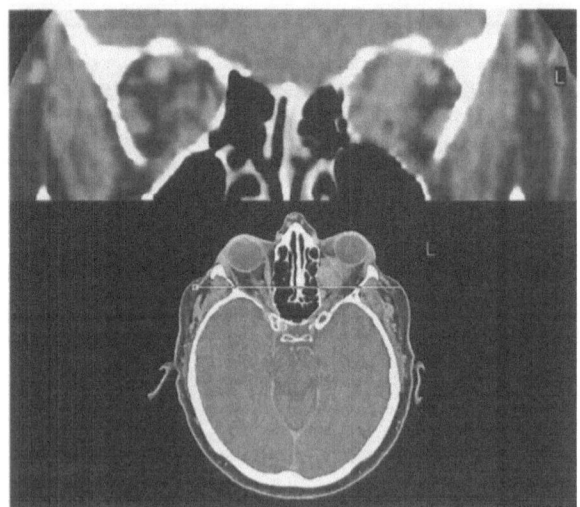

10.6

CT
Large, roundish, space-occupying lesion in the superior and medial intraconal space. The lamina papyracea is impressed, the globe is displaced anteriorly. Enlargement of the superior ophthalmic veins, convolutions of small orbital veins.

Diagnosis
Venous malformation.

Comment
The impression of the lamina papyracea is suggestive of a longstanding tumor.

Plate 6

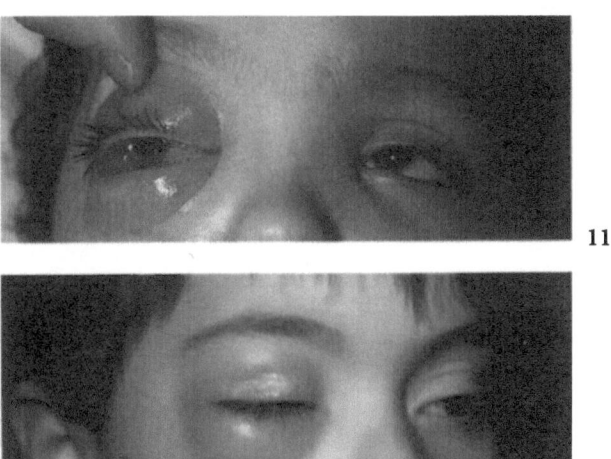

11

12

Both children exhibit complete ptosis, massive periorbital swelling and hyperemia, as well as chemosis.

T. D., 4-year-old girl

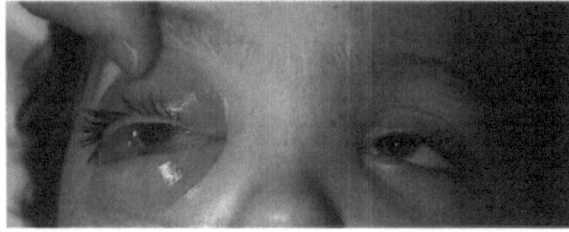

11.1

History and Clinical Findings
Rapidly increasing periorbital swelling, proptosis, restricted ocular motility, and chemosis for the past few days.

Diagnosis
Panophthalmitis.

K. V., 4-year-old boy

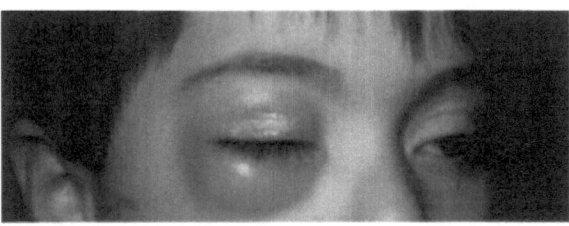

12.1

History and Clinical Findings
Head injury and subsequent slight periorbital swelling 1 week ago. Now sudden increase of periorbital swelling and hyperemia. Upper respiratory tract infection and fever. No laboratory signs of infection.

CT
Partial opacification of the maxillary sinuses, the ethmoidal air cells, and the sphenoid sinuses. Frac-

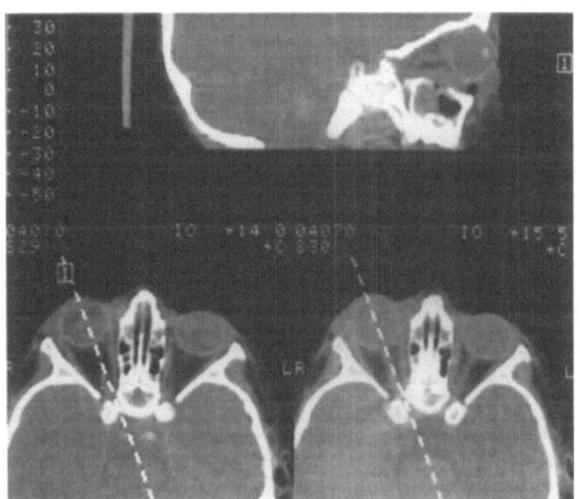

12.2

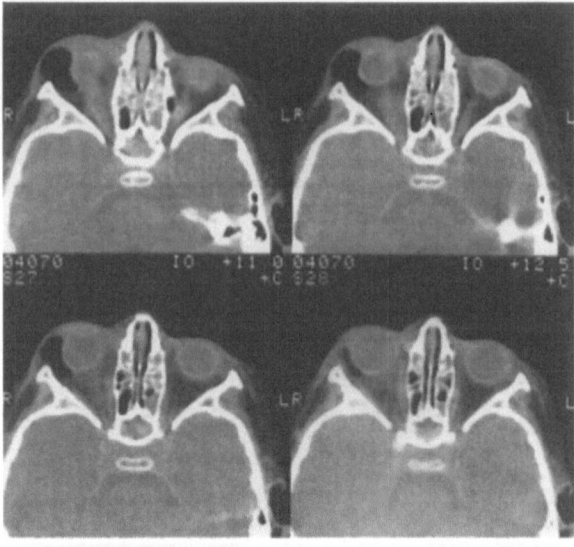

12.3

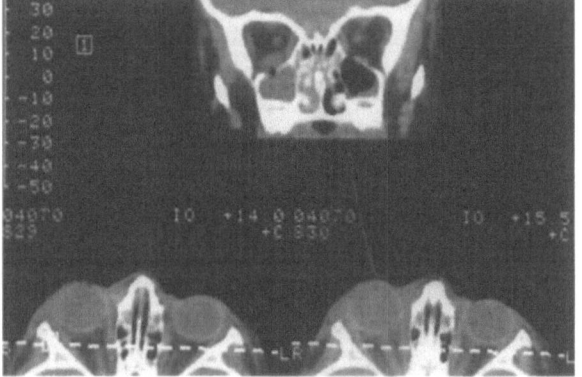

12.4

ture of the right orbital floor. Air within the inferior and lateral extraconal space. Hyperdense areas within the inferior extraconal space. Protrusion of the right globe.

Diagnosis
Fracture of the orbital floor with air emphysema and a hematoma within the inferior extraconal space.

Clinical Course
Complete remission with no surgical or medical treatment.

Comment
With no knowledge of the history of trauma, which children might keep secret if brought about by forbidden activities, the clinical findings might suggest the diagnosis of orbital cellulitis. Visualisation of the broken orbital floor and the large amount of air within the orbital space allows differentiation from bacterial sinusitis caused by gas-producing bacteria.

Plate 7

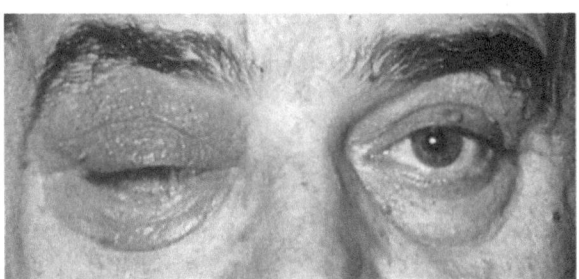

13

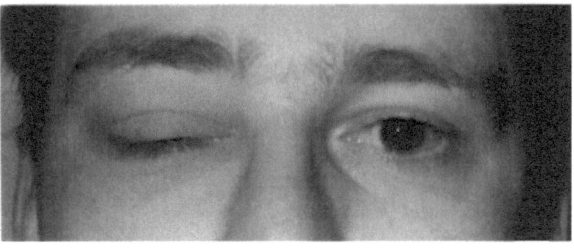

14

Both patients exhibit ptosis as well as periorbital
swelling and hyperemia.

K. H., 52-year-old man

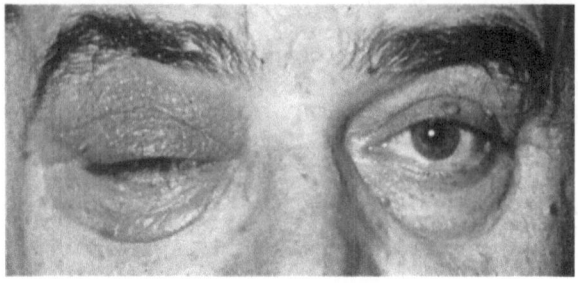

13.1

History and Clinical Findings
Acute onset of periorbital swelling and hyperemia. Decreased visual acuity and severe headaches. Uveitis.

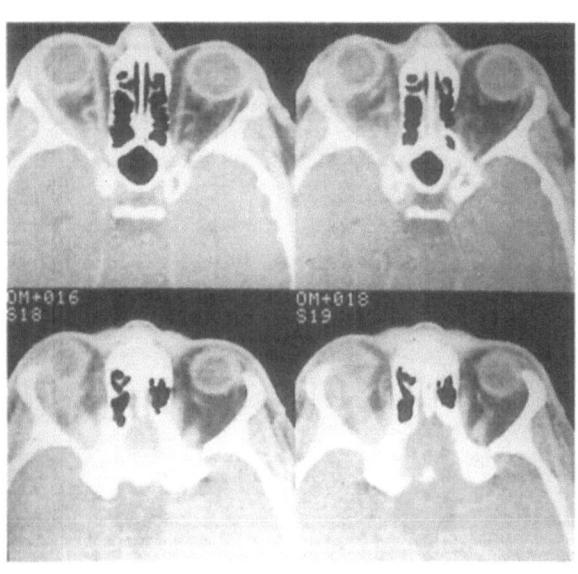

13.2

CT
Diffuse infiltration of the lateral half of the right orbit. Enlargement of the lateral rectus muscle including its tendon, as well as of the wall of the globe. Slight enlargement of the lacrimal gland.

Diagnosis
Diffuse infiltration of the orbit, myositis, tendonitis, scleritis-tenonitis, and concomitant dacryoadenitis: inflammatory orbital pseudotumor.

Clinical Course
Complete remission of symptoms after steroid treatment (beginning with 100 mg prednisolone, slowly and gradually reducing the dose).

K. M., 30-year-old man

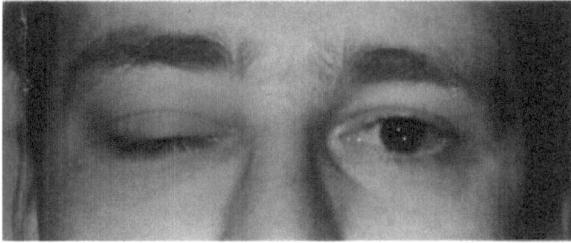

14.1

History and Clinical Findings
X-ray of the sinuses 14 days ago: complete opacification of the right maxillary sinus. Right hemicephalgia and pain in the right jaw, both increasing in intensity over the past few days. Systemic antibiotic treatment.

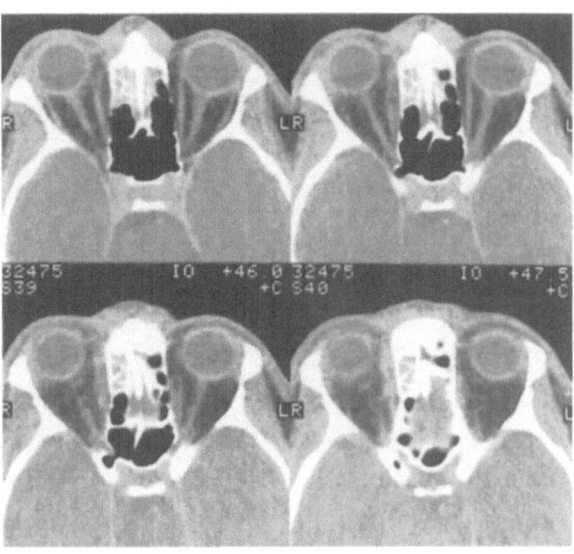

14.4

Swelling of the right upper lid for 3 days. Ipsilateral ptosis and proptosis, as well as restriction of upward gaze for 2 days.

CT
Hyperdense areas in the right maxillary sinus and in the right ethmoidal air cells. Defects in the lamina papyracea. Soft-tissue swelling near the right upper lid. Enlargement of the right superior oblique muscle. Inhomogeneous areas of increased density within the adjacent extraconal space.

Diagnosis
Acute sinusitis of the maxillary sinus and of the ethmoidal air cells. Defects in the lamina papyracea. Subperiosteal abscess. Concomitant myositis of the right superior oblique muscle.

Clinical Course
Sinus lavage and systemic antibiotic treatment. Complete remission of signs and symptoms within 12 days.

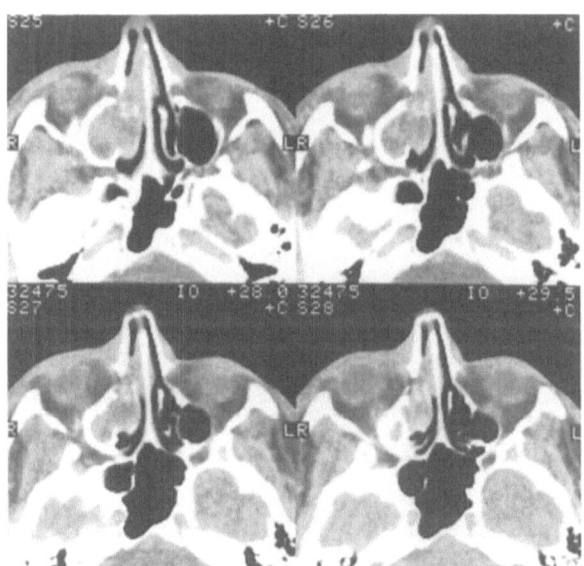

14.2

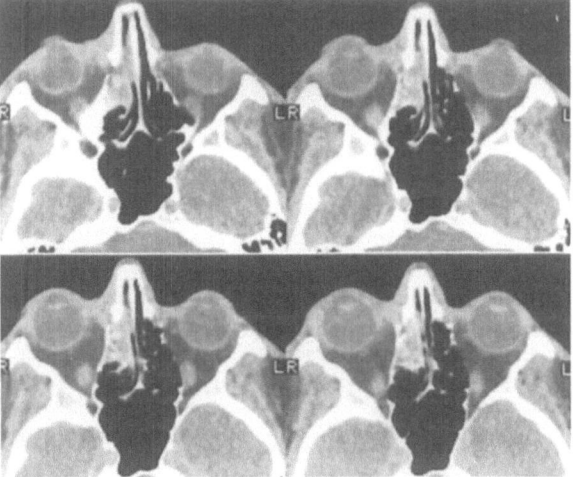

14.3

Plate 8

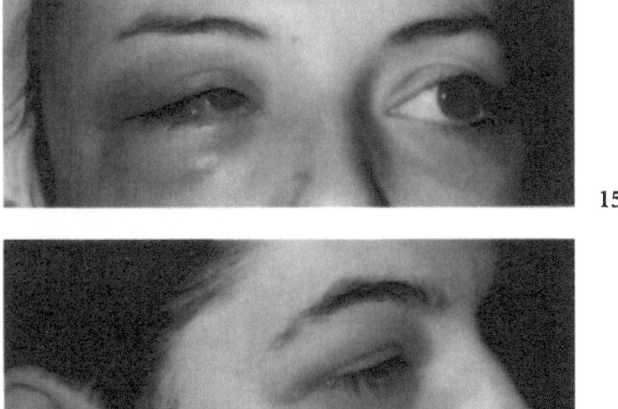

15

16

Both patients exhibit massive unilateral periorbital
swelling and hyperemia, as well as chemosis.

R. P., 29-year-old woman

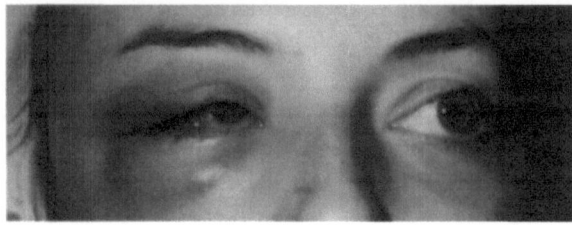

15.1

History and Clinical Findings
Large abscess within the right cheek which had
been incised and drained.

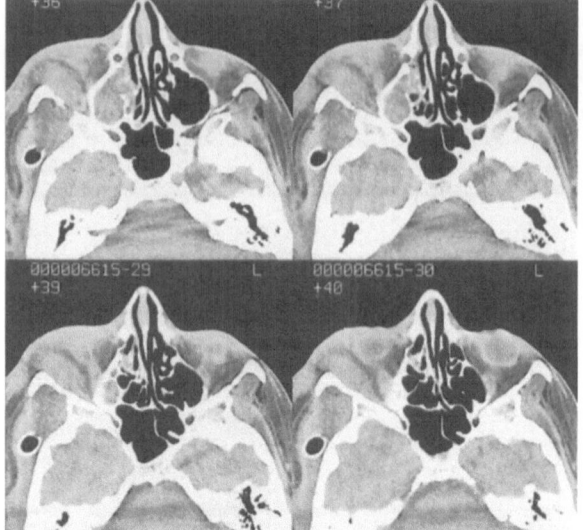

15.2

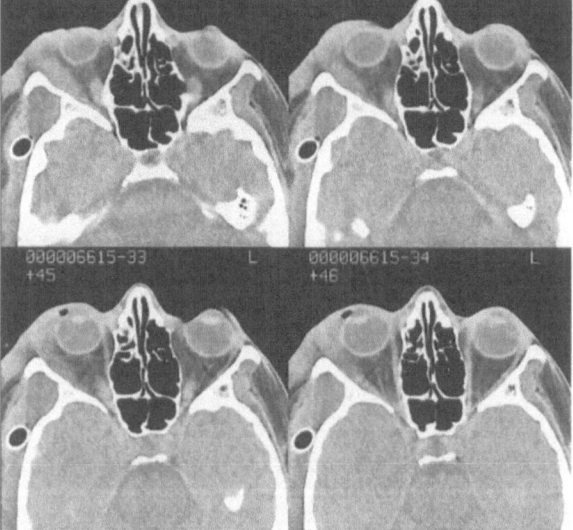

15.3

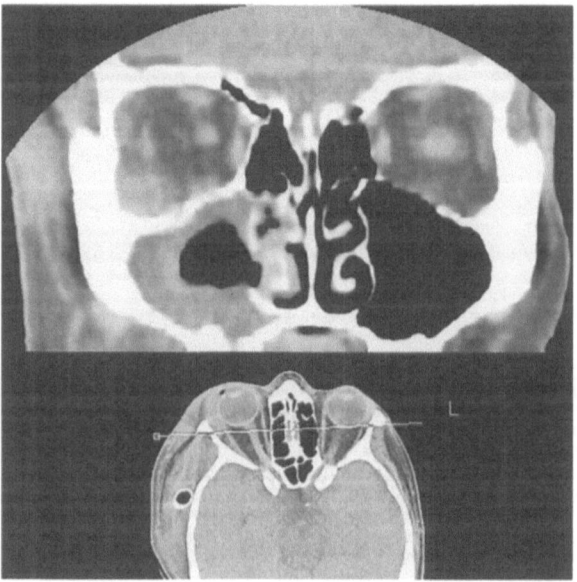

(Continued on p. 33)

15.4

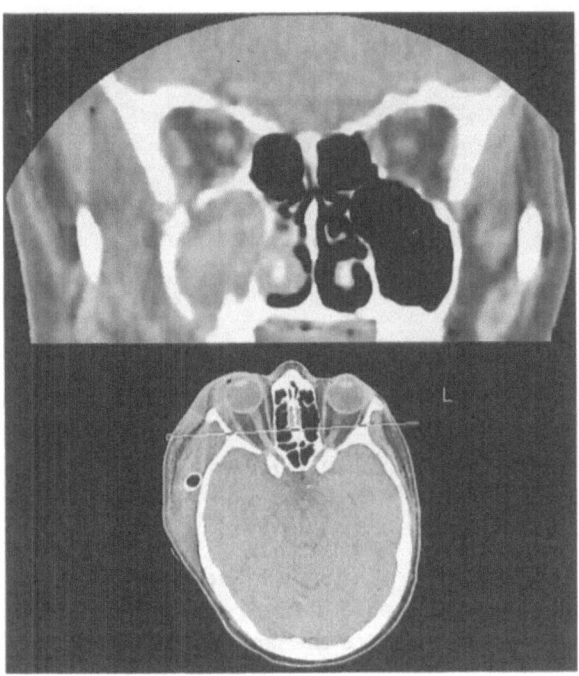

15.5

CT

Diffuse infiltration of the right retro-maxillary space and the cheek. Spontaneous drainage via the retro-maxillary space. Air-fluid level in the right maxillary sinus and numerous bone defects. Enlargement of the right lateral rectus muscle and the right lacrimal gland. Infiltration of the lateral extraconal space.

Diagnosis

Abscess-forming inflammation in the right retro-maxillary space and the cheek. Sinusitis of the maxillary sinus causing bone destruction. Infiltration of the lateral extraconal space. Concomitant inflammation of the right lateral rectus muscle and concomitant dacryoadenitis.

P. R., 23-year-old man

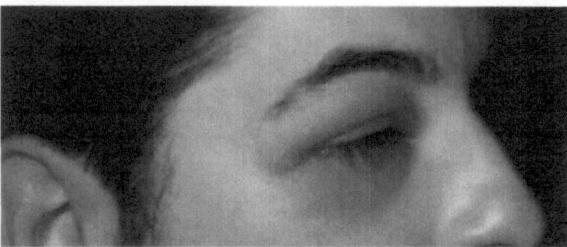

16.1

History and Clinical Findings
According to the patient, optic neuritis had been diagnosed and treated with steroids. Recurrence of signs and symptoms after discontinuation of therapy.

    Presently, self-medication with steroids.

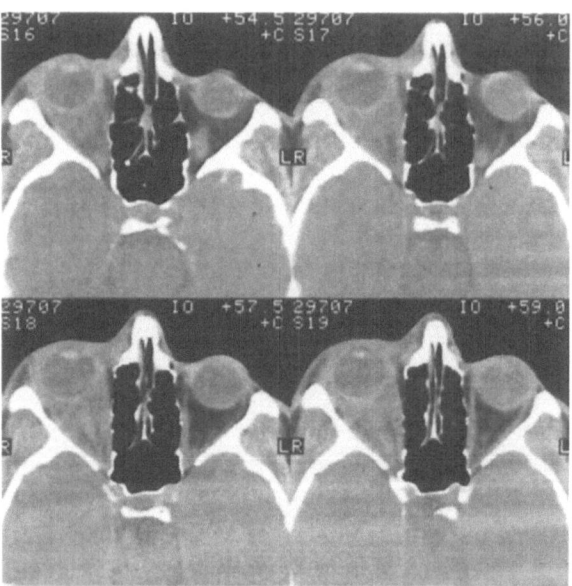

16.2

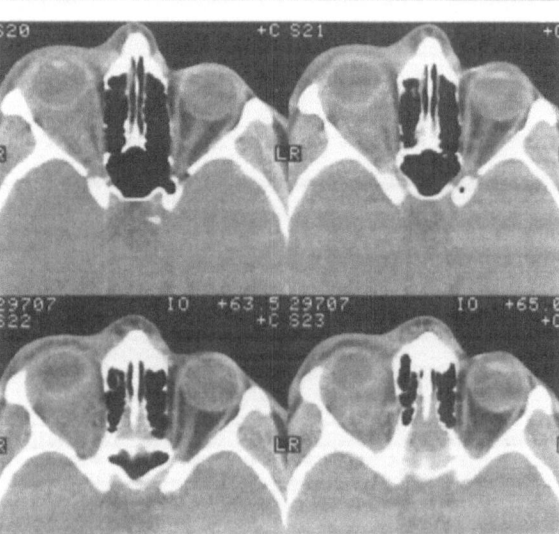

16.3

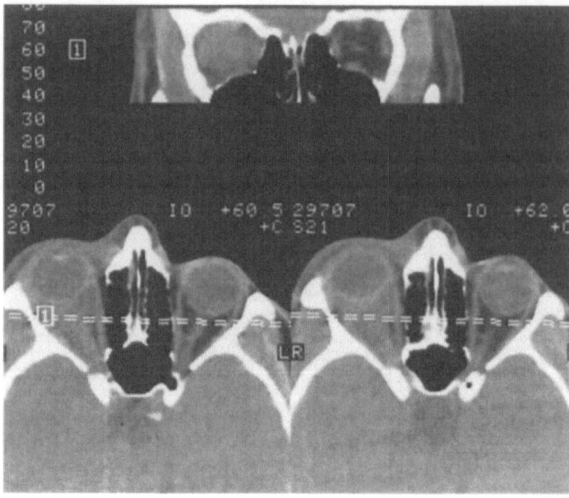

16.4

CT
Extended areas of increased density within the right intraconal space. Tenon's capsule is enlarged. Slight enlargement of the lacrimal gland. Infiltration of the right lid. Protrusion of the globe. The paranasal sinuses are normal.

Diagnosis
Diffusely infiltrating form of inflammatory orbital pseudotumor. Systemic disease must be excluded.

Clinical Course
Remission of signs and symptoms with steroid treatment (beginning with 100 mg prednisolone, slowly and gradually reducing the dose). Systemic disease was excluded.

Plate 9

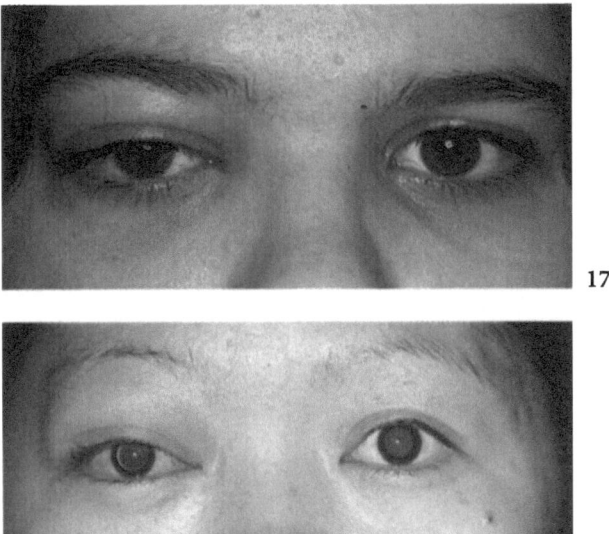

17

18

Both patients exhibit swelling of the upper lid, moderate ptosis, and episcleral venous injection.

F. C., 15-year-old girl

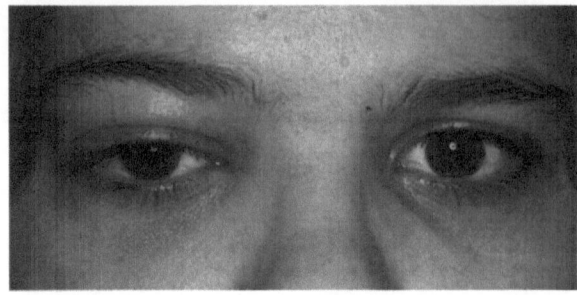

17.1

History and Clinical Findings
Increasing swelling and hyperemia of the right upper lid for a few days. Episcleral venous injection. Severe pain.

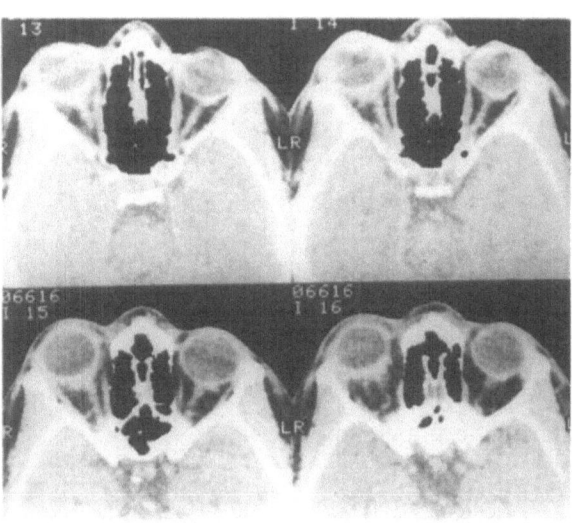

17.2

CT
Considerable enlargement of the wall of the globe. Slight infiltration of the retrobulbar space.

Diagnosis
Scleritic-tenonitic form of inflammatory orbital pseudotumor.

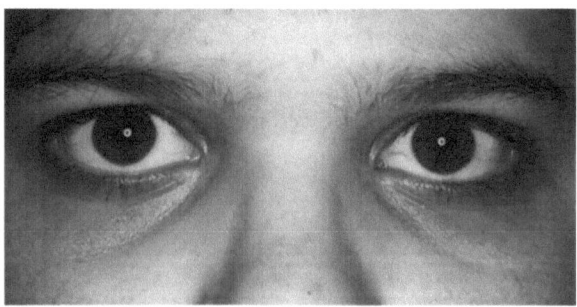

17.3

Clinical aspect after a 7-day course of steroids (17.3).

H.K., 40-year-old woman

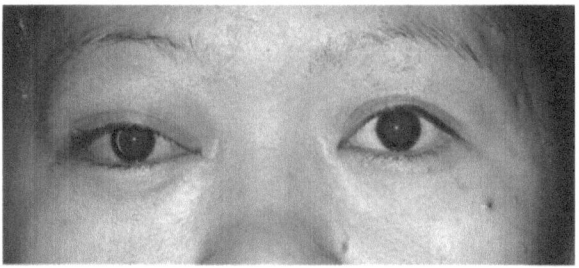

18.1

History and Clinical Findings
Severe head injury 2 months ago. Increasing swelling of the right upper lid, ptosis, and episcleral venous injection.

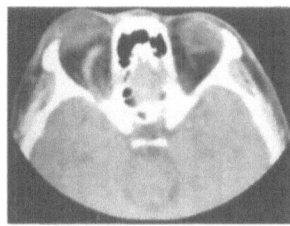

18.2

CT
Massive enlargement of the right superior ophthalmic vein.

Diagnosis
Posttraumatic fistula between the carotid artery and the cavernous sinus.

Case courtesy of Professor T.H. Newton, former Chief of Neuroradiology, Department of Radiology, University of California Medical School, San Francisco, California, USA.

Plate 10

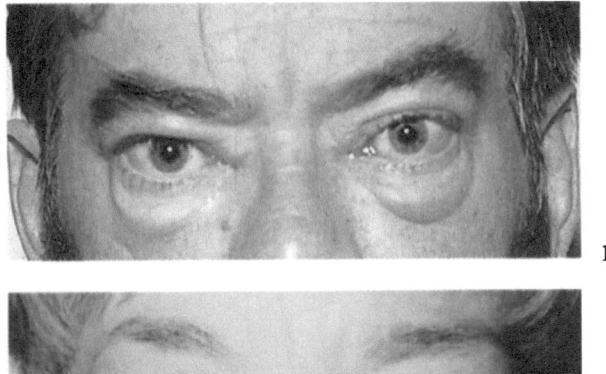

19

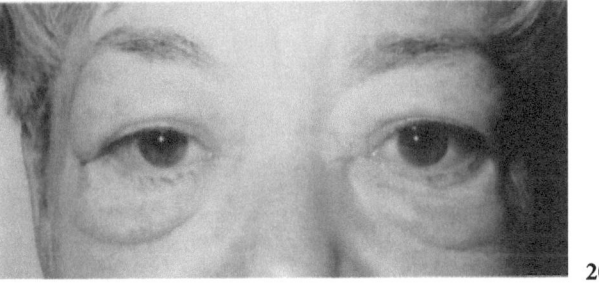

20

Both patients exhibit bilateral chemosis and doughy
periorbital swelling.

J. H.-W., 50-year-old man

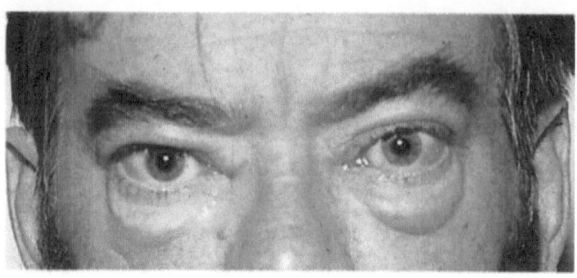

19.1

History and Clinical Findings
Slowly progressive periorbital swelling and chemosis for 3 weeks.

CT (not shown)
Bilaterally, slight, diffuse infiltration of extraocular
muscles and of the orbital fat.

Diagnosis
Low-grade non-Hodgkin lymphoma.
Thyroid disease was excluded.

P.R., 62-year-old woman

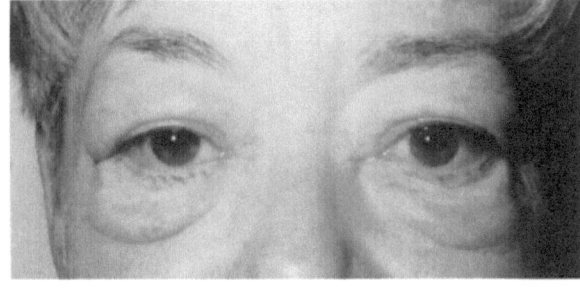

20.1

History and Clinical Findings

Hyperthyroidism was diagnosed 6 months ago. Antithyroid medication, presently euthyroid.

At present, swelling of the temporal parts of both upper lids, and massive swelling of both lower lids. Chemosis. Bilaterally, slight restriction of upward gaze.

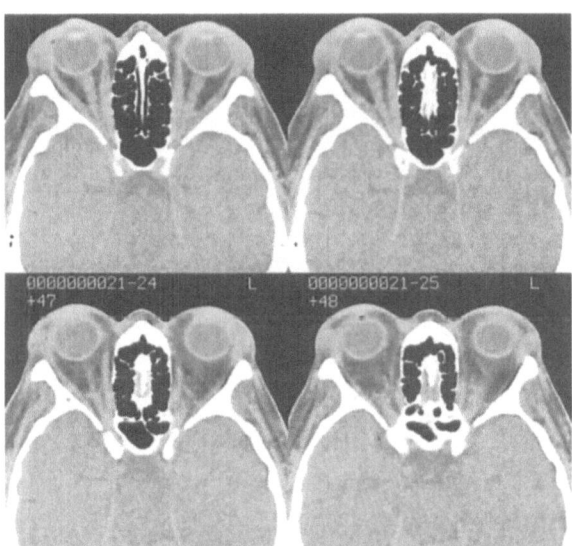

20.2

20.3
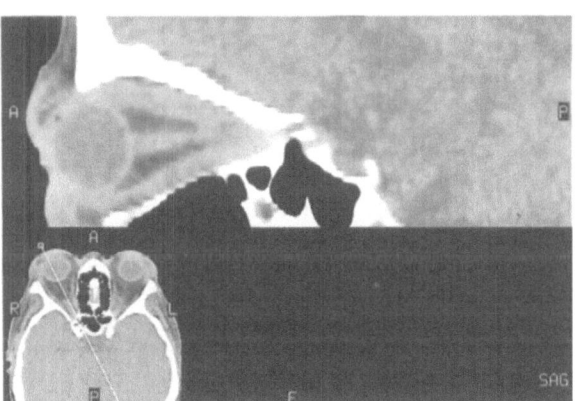

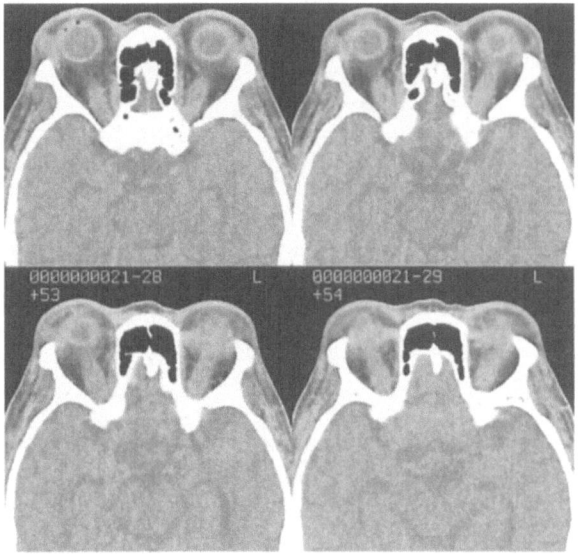

20.4

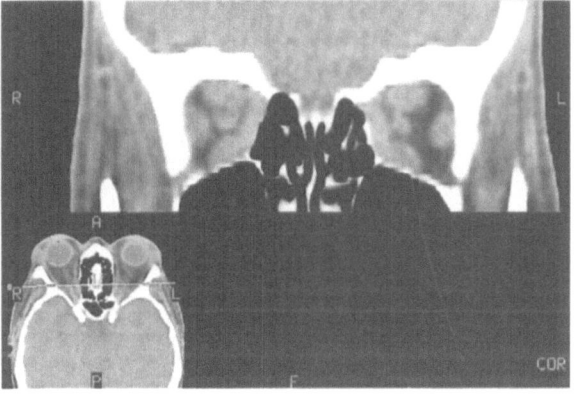

20.5

CT

Considerable enlargement of most extraocular muscles. Increase in the volume of the orbital fat and protrusion of both globes. Slight enlargement and forward displacement of the palpebral portion of the lacrimal gland. Lid swelling.

Diagnosis

Polymyositic form of Graves' disease.

Plate 11

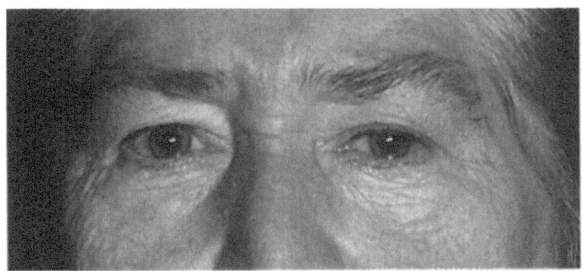

21

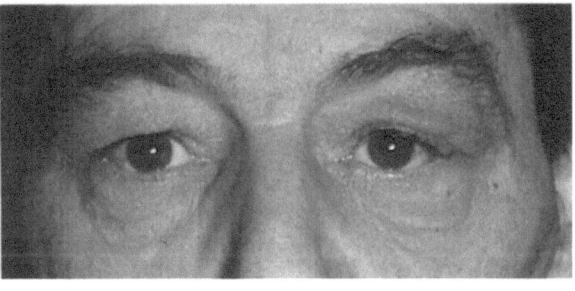

22

Both patients exhibit unilateral swelling of the
upper lid and slight hyperemia of the temporal
upper lid.

K. M., 65-year-old woman

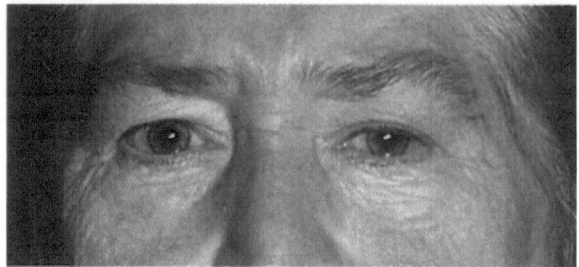

21.1

History and Clinical Findings
Swelling and hyperemia of the left upper lid and pain for 3 weeks.

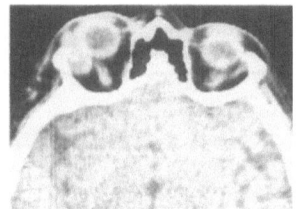

21.2

CT
Considerable enlargement of the right lacrimal gland with irregular, hypodense areas.

Diagnosis
Dacryoadenitis with abscess formation.

Clinical Course
Spontaneous drainage. Systemic antibiotic treatment followed by complete remission.

S. H., 56-year-old man

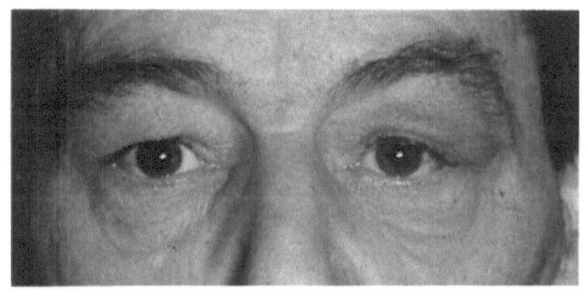

22.1

History and Clinical Findings
Painless swelling of the lateral left upper lid. Protrusion of the palpebral portion of the lacrimal gland.

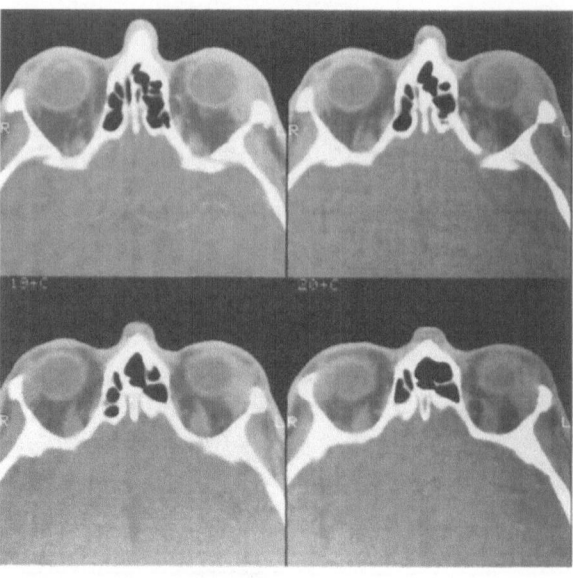

22.2

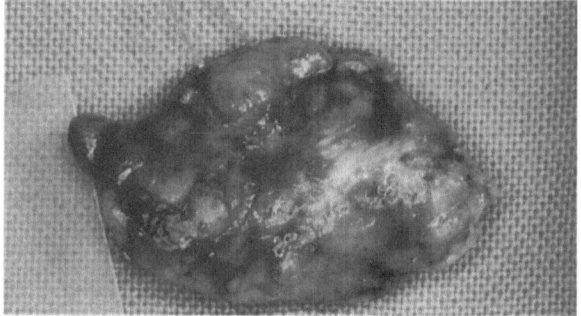

22.3

CT
Homogeneous enlargement of the lacrimal gland nestling closely against the globe, extending into the retrobulbar space without impressing the globe.

Differential Diagnosis
Unspecific inflammation or neoplastic infiltration.

Clinical Course
Lateral orbitotomy with removal of the left lacrimal gland.

Histopathology
Chronic, scarring and sclerosing dacryoadenitis. Since this form of dacryoadenitis may be caused by pathological immune reactions, another thorough medical examination was indicated. This yielded no indication of any autoimmune disease.

Comment
In this case, a biopsy of the lacrimal gland would have been sufficient because the enlargement was homogeneous and no signs of systemic inflammatory or neoplastic disease were found.

Plate 12

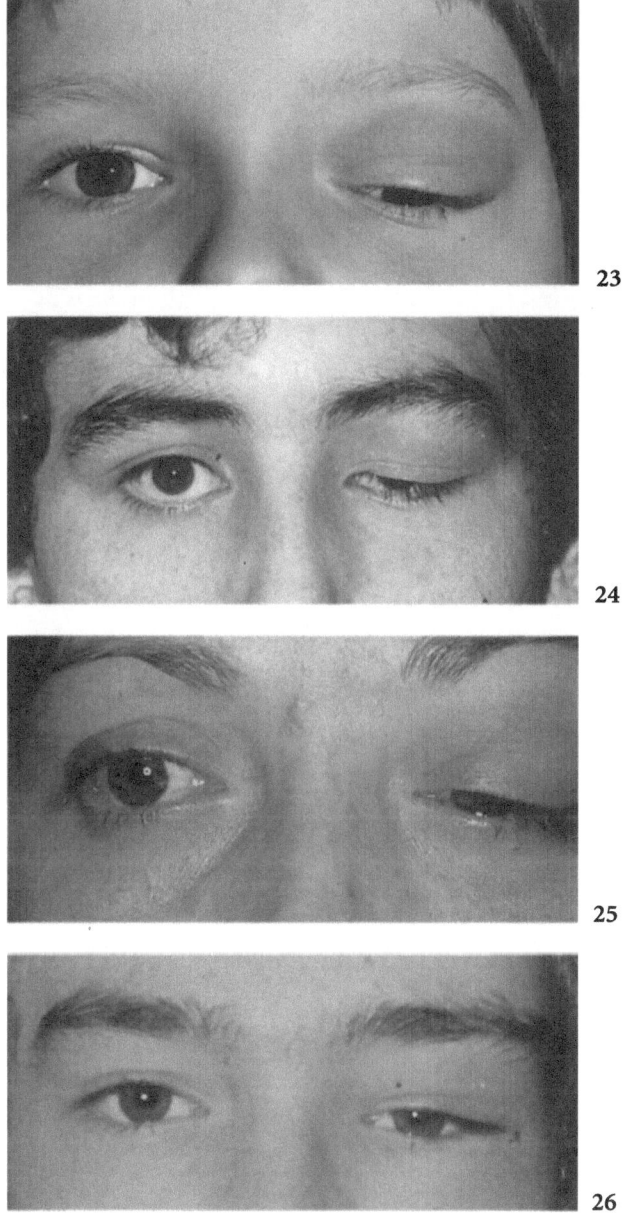

23

24

25

26

All four patients exhibit unilateral ptosis and temporally accentuated swelling of the upper lid, which developed within 7 days.

Case 23: 12-year-old boy
Diagnosis: Neuroblastoma.

Case 24: 16-year-old boy
Diagnosis: Subperiosteal abscess.

Case 25: 26-year-old woman
Diagnosis: Dacryoadenitic form of inflammatory orbital pseudotumor.

Case 26: 14-year-old boy
Diagnosis: Histiocytosis X (see Case 72).

Different Aspects of Eight Patients with Clinically Proven Graves' Disease

Plate 13

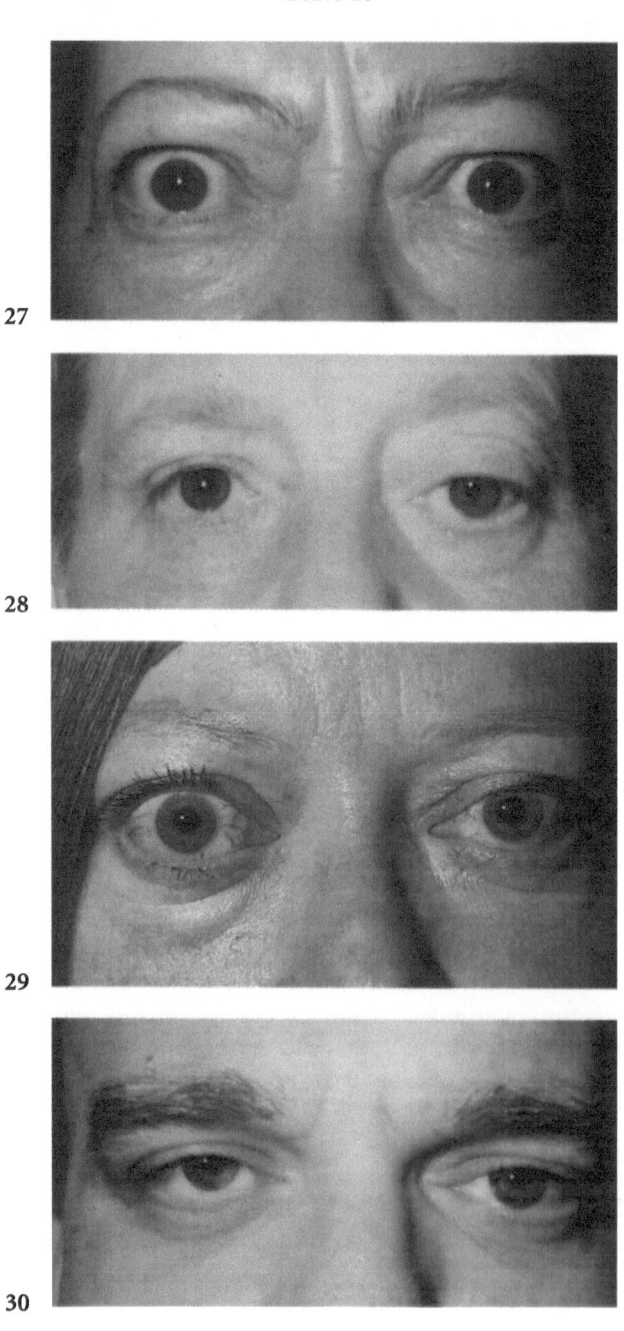

27

28

29

30

Plate 14

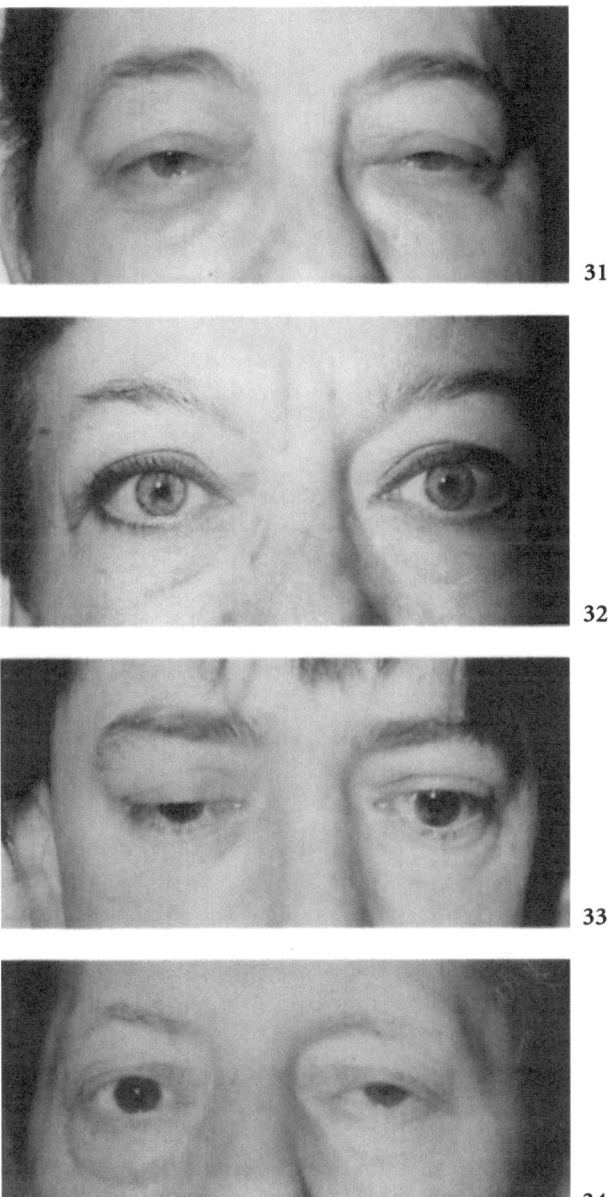

V. C., 52-year-old woman

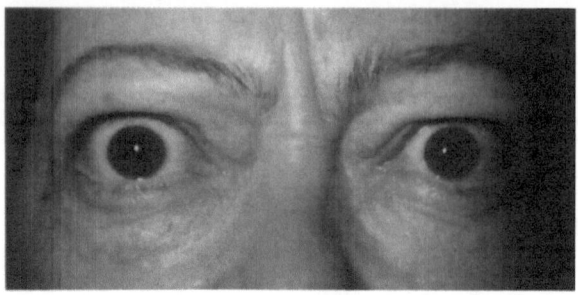

27.1

History and Clinical Findings

Ten years ago, the patient was diagnosed with Graves' disease and treated by near-total thyroidectomy. At present she does not take any medication.

Bilaterally, restriction of upward gaze and of abduction. Bilateral proptosis, lid retraction and periorbital swelling, more pronounced on the right side.

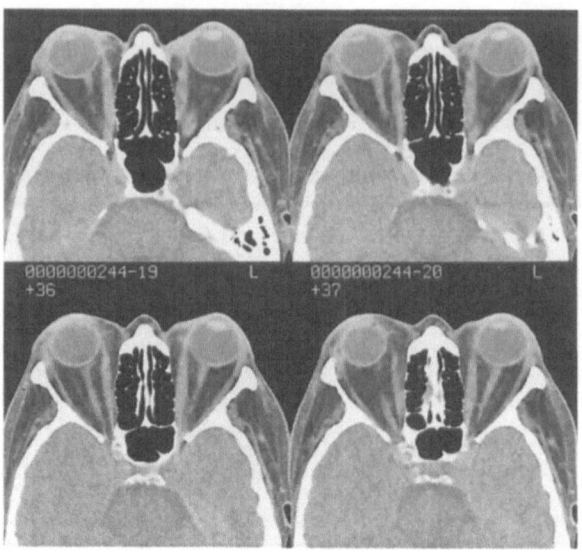

27.2

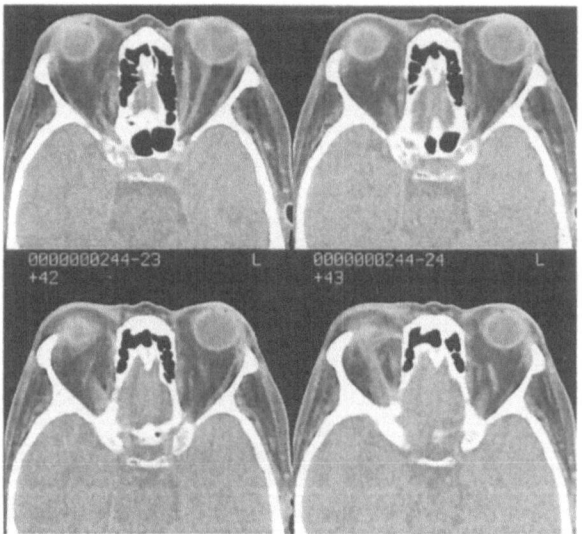

27.3

CT

Moderate enlargement of most extraocular muscles, particularly of the upper muscle complex and of the inferior and medial rectus muscles. Small, hypodense areas in some muscles, suggestive of fibrotic transformation. Considerable increase in the volume of the orbital fat.

Diagnosis

Polymyositic form of Graves' disease. Partial fibrotic transformation.

Comment

Muscle enlargement is moderate. Pronounced proptosis is predominantly caused by the increase in the volume of the orbital fat.

J. K., 53-year-old woman

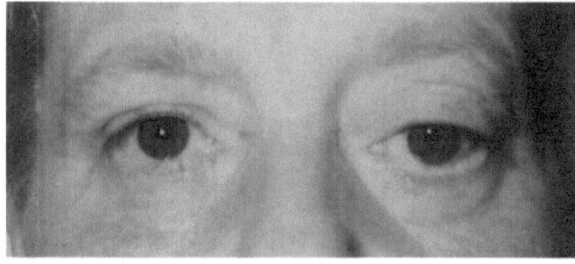

28.1

History and Clinical Findings
Protrusion of the left globe and diplopia for the past 9 years.

The patient underwent radiation therapy and steroid treatment for Graves' disease. Ocular muscle surgery scheduled.

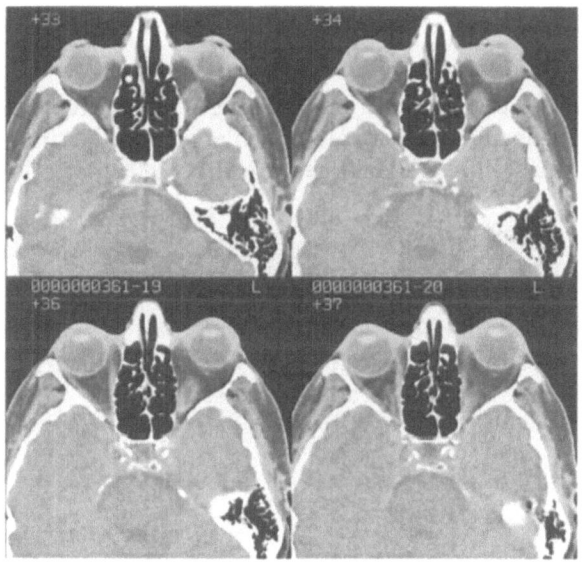

28.2

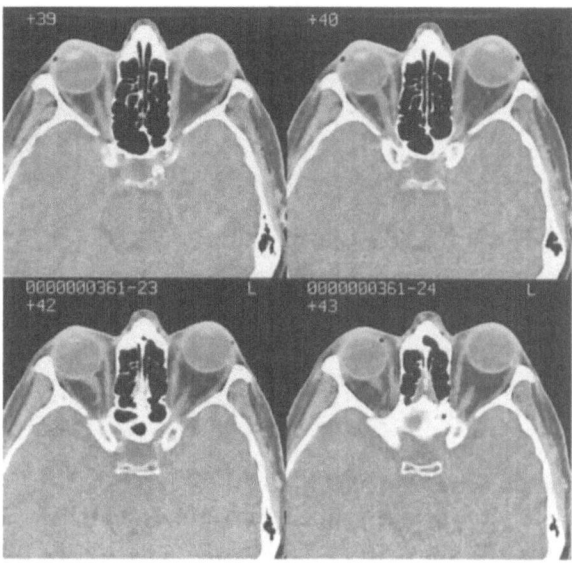

28.3

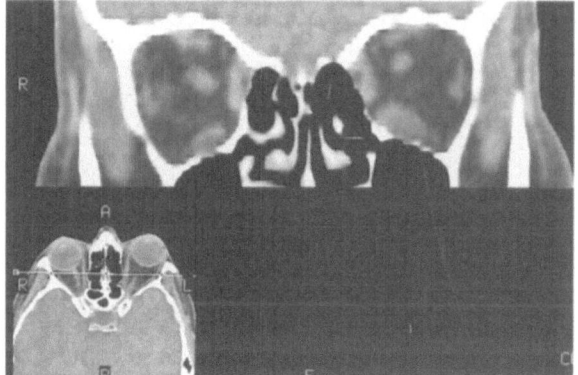

28.4

CT
Enlargement of the left inferior rectus muscle. Small, hypodense areas within the muscle. Protrusion of the left globe and increase in the volume of the orbital fat.

Diagnosis
Monomyositic form of Graves' disease: "inferior rectus muscle syndrome". Partial fibrotic transformation.

Comment
The clinical aspect is suggestive of a neoplasm rather than of Graves' disease.
Ptosis is obviously due to a myopathy of the levator palpebrae muscle.

J. G., 47-year-old woman

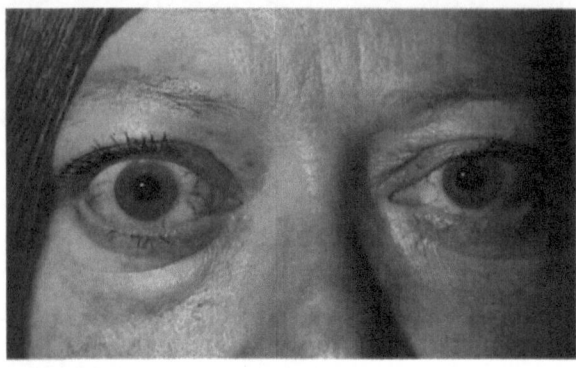

29.1

History and Clinical Findings
The patient takes antithyroid medication and is presently euthyroid.

Increasing proptosis and lid retraction on the right side.

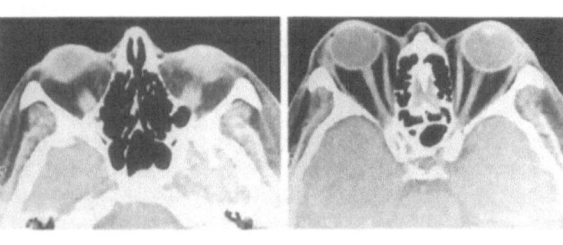

9.2–3

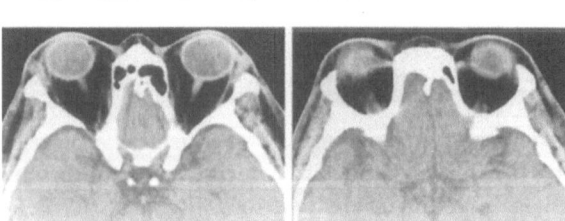

9.4–5

CT
Massive increase in the volume of the orbital fat. Extraocular muscles are not enlarged. The lacrimal glands, while not enlarged, are displaced anteriorly.

Diagnosis
Graves' disease.

Clinical Course
Hyperthyroid episode 18 months later. Enlargement of several extraocular muscles.

S.W., 40-year-old man

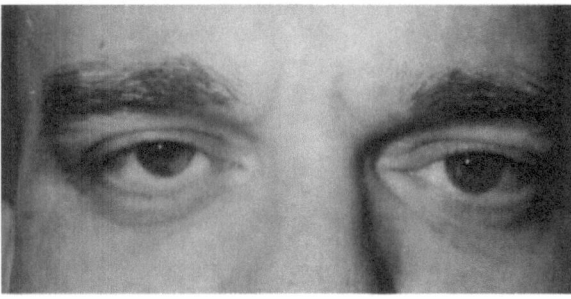

30.1

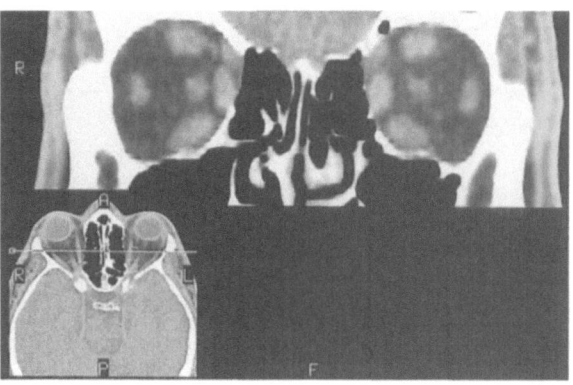

30.3

History and Clinical Findings
Five months ago hyperthyroidism was diagnosed. Thyroid-related antibodies were elevated. The patient takes antithyroid medication.

Hyperlacrimation, periorbital hyperemia, photophobia, and pain for two months.

CT
Slight enlargement of several extraocular muscles with small, hypodense areas. The orbital septum is slightly bulged out. The lacrimal gland is slightly enlarged.

Diagnosis
Polymyositic form of Graves' disease. The hypodense areas are suggestive of fibrotic transformation.

Comment
Since ptosis is bilateral, the patient should be tested for acetylcholine receptor antibodies to exclude myasthenia (Vargas et al. 1993).

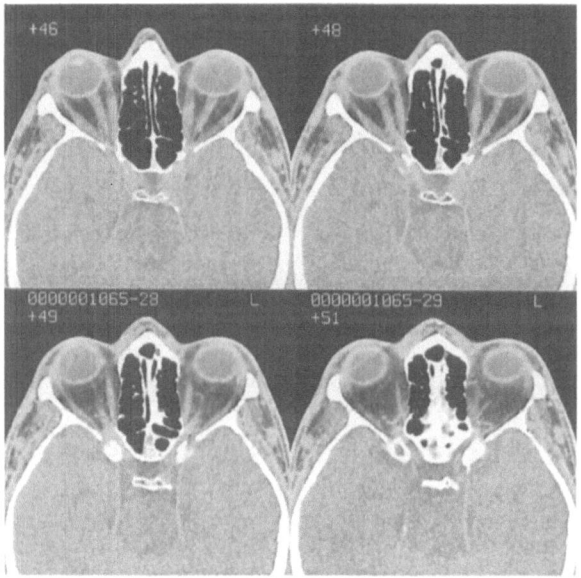

30.2

B. H.-W., 60-year-old man

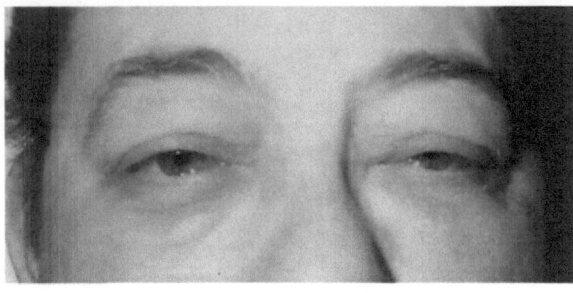

31.1

History and Clinical Findings
Bilaterally, progressive restriction of upward gaze and of abduction.
   Steroid treatment was ineffective.

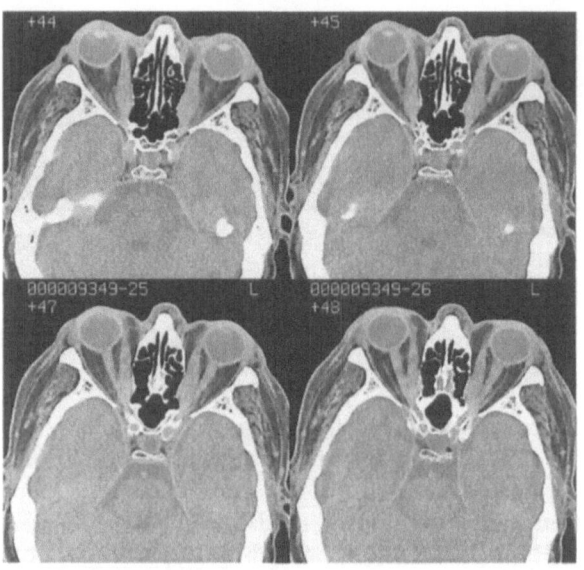

31.3

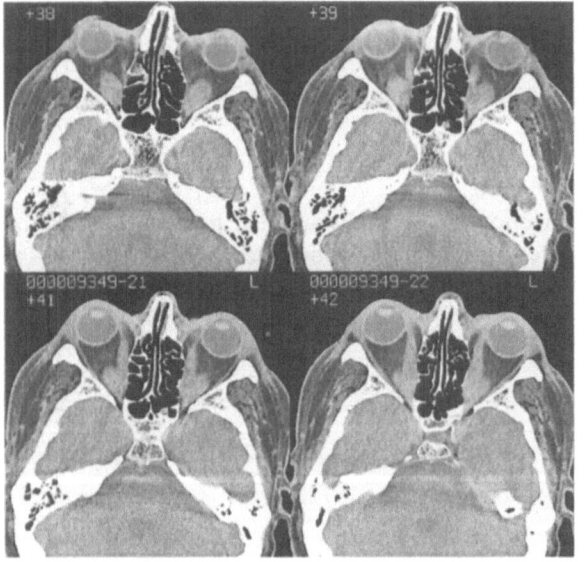

31.2

CT
Considerable enlargement of several extraocular muscles with small, hypodense areas indicating partial fibrotic transformation. Protrusion of the globe and increase in the volume of the orbital fat.

Diagnosis
Polymyositic form of Graves' disease.

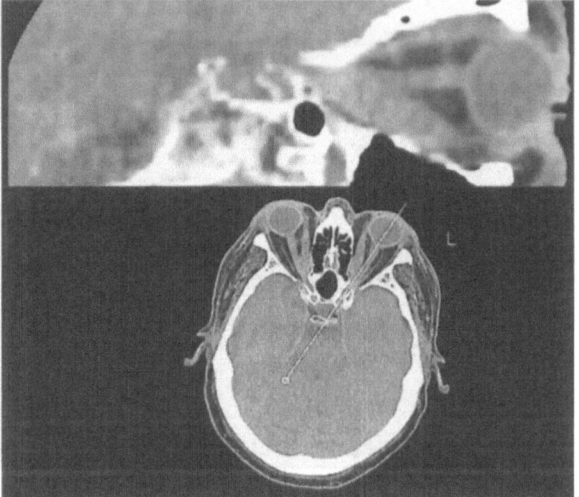

31.4

Clinical Course
Remission of clinical signs and symptoms after therapeutic radiation of the orbital apex.

Comment
Due to the relatively tight orbital septum, proptosis is only moderate. Since ptosis is bilateral, the patient should be tested for acetylcholine receptor antibodies to exclude associated myasthenia.

K. R., 49-year-old woman

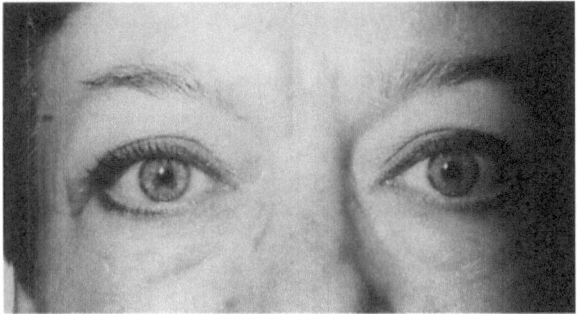

32.1

History and Clinical Findings
Hyperthyroidism and proptosis diagnosed 2 years ago. Antithyroid medication for 3 months, subsequently, near-total thyroidectomy. Double vision for 4 weeks.

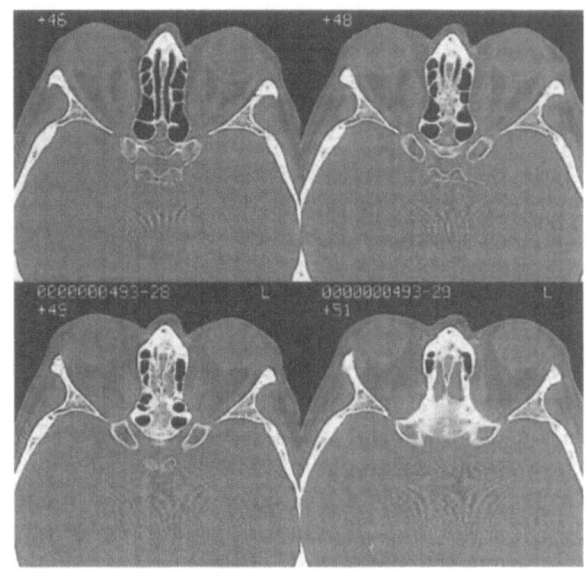

32.3

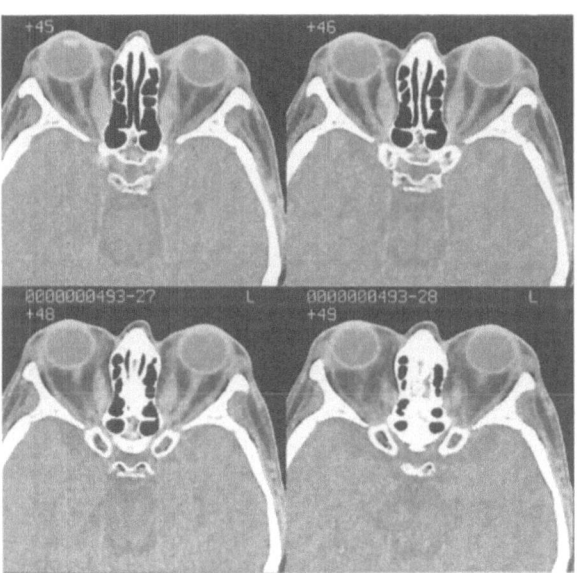

32.2

CT
Considerable enlargement of most extraocular muscles. Slight increase in the volume of the orbital fat. Bilateral proptosis. Bilateral impression of the lamina papyracea ("Coca-Cola bottle sign").

Diagnosis
Polymyositic form of Graves' disease.

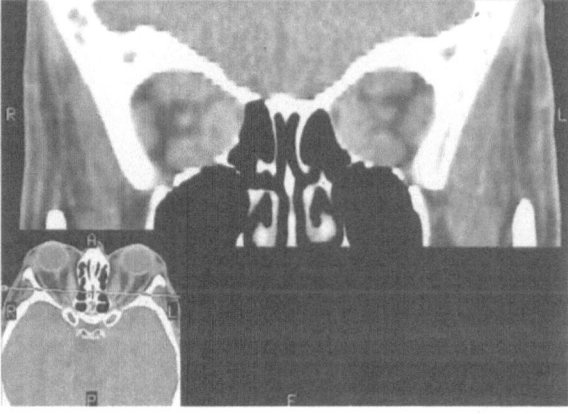

32.4

Comment
The striking disparity between the very slight proptosis without lid retraction and the considerable muscle enlargement is probably due to the increase in intraorbital space, caused by the deformation and displacement of the lamina papyracea.

F. U., 35-year-old man

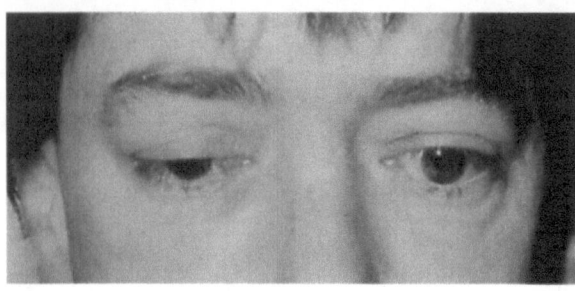

33.1

History and Clinical Findings

Ptosis of unknown origin for the past 7 years. The patient was diagnosed with hyperthyroidism 6 months ago, and was placed on antithyroid medication. Endocrine ophthalmopathy and infiltration of both the palpebral and orbital portion of the right lacrimal gland was suspected.

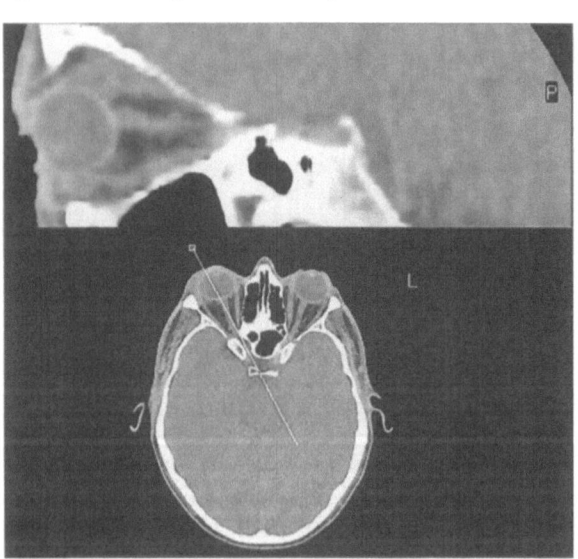

33.2

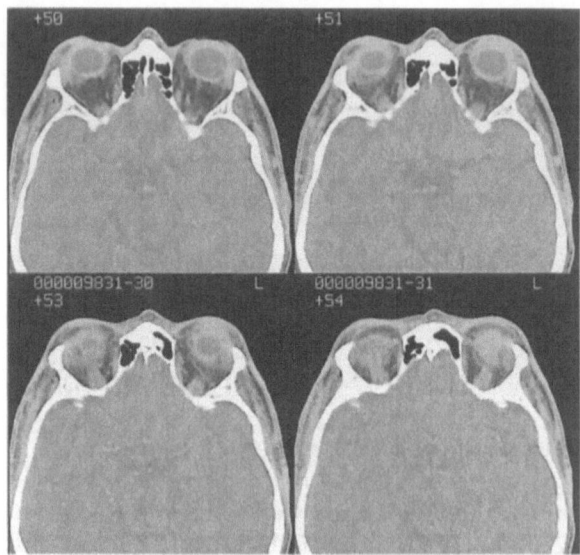

33.3

33.4

CT

Bilaterally, considerable enlargement of the upper muscle complex. Slight enlargement of both lacrimal glands. Swelling of the lids.

Diagnosis

Polymyositic form of Graves' disease with concomitant dacryoadenitis.

R. W., 53-year-old woman

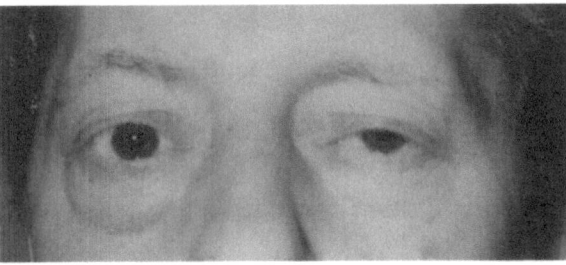

34.1

History and Clinical Findings

Protrusion of the right globe was first noticed 7 years ago; the patient was then diagnosed with a thyroid disorder.

Presentation for *enophthalmos* on the left side.

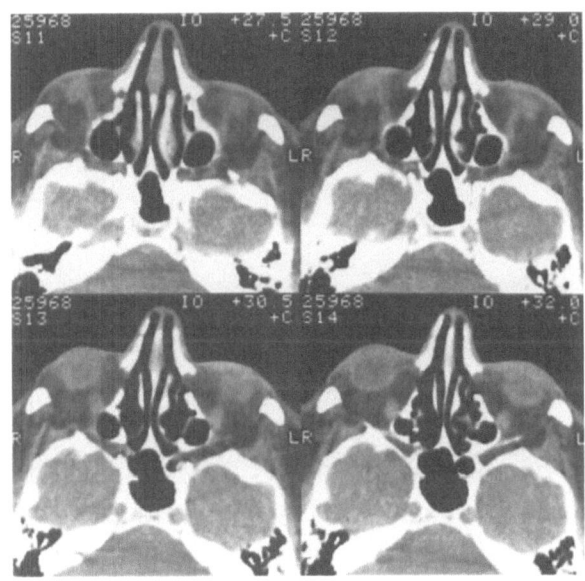

34.2

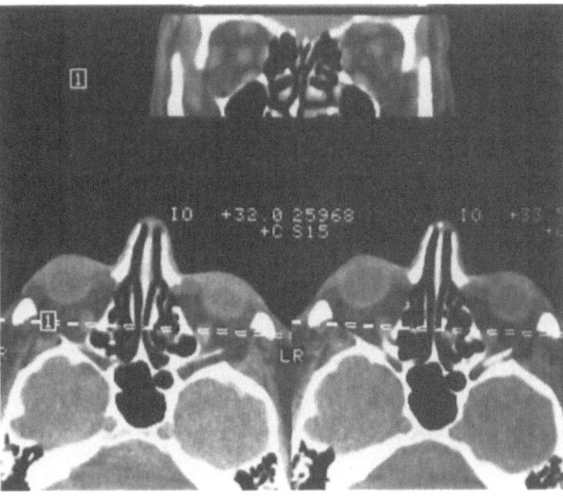

34.3

CT

Protrusion of the right globe. The orbital septum is bulged out due to an increase in the volume of the orbital fat. Large bone defect in the posterior and inferior lateral orbital wall with herniation of orbital fat. The more extensive decompression on the left side causes the left eye to appear enophthalmic.

Diagnosis

Graves' ophthalmopathy and spontaneous decompression.

Comment

There are no signs of either muscle infiltration or fibrotic transformation.

The longstanding increase in orbital pressure has led to bone erosions.

3 Graves' Disease

Definition and Pathogenesis

Orbital Graves' disease is an inflammatory disease of the orbital tissues associated with an immune thyroiditis, most often with hyperthyroidism of the Basedow type, less commonly with Hashimoto's thyroiditis. It is the most common orbital disease in adults. Orbital signs and symptoms usually occur simultaneously with the thyroid disorder, but sometimes months or even years earlier or later. The relationship between the thyroid and the orbital disease has not yet been fully investigated. Thyroid hormone secretion does not seem to be a decisive factor in the course of Graves' disease. Changes in the course of this disease, either worsening or improvement, following therapy with radioactive iodine or near-total thyroidectomy are considered to indicate that released thyroid antigens shift the antigen-antibody ratio. This assumption is substantiated by the fact that the worsening of Graves' disease following radioactive iodine administration can, in many cases, be successfully suppressed by steroid therapy (Bartalena et al. 1989).

The broad clinical spectrum of Graves' disease and the variety of clinical manifestations, of responses to different therapeutic measures, and of laboratory findings and CT patterns indicates that what we currently refer to as Graves' disease is probably a group of heterogeneous disorders. The association of Graves' disease with HLA types B8, BW35, DR3, and subtype DW3, which are also associated with other immunological diseases, for example myasthenia gravis, diabetes type I, and pernicious anemia, points to a genetic predisposition. In patients suffering from Graves' disease, other signs of disordered immune regulation, such as thymus hyperplasia, lymphadenopathy, or splenomegaly, may be seen. Patients with Graves' disease may produce various autoantibodies: thyroid-stimulating-hormone receptor antibodies, microsomal antibodies, i.e., antibodies against thyroid peroxidase, and thyroglobulin antibodies. Some antibodies stimulate, while others inhibit thyroid function. Antinuclear and antimitochondrial antibodies are found with higher frequency in patients with Graves' disease. Regarding the autoimmune pathogenesis, cross-immunity of antibodies to bacterial and viral antigens ("molecular mimicry"), analogies between thyroglobulin and acetyl cholinesterase, and increased antigen expression on thyrocytes stimulated by interferon-γ have been discussed.

The initial stage of Graves' disease is caused by lymphoplasmacellular infiltration. One possible explanation is that circulating T-cells, directed against a thyrocyte antigen, recognize the same antigen on orbital fibroblasts. T-cells infiltrate orbital tissues and induce fibroblast proliferation. Cytokines, such as INF-γ, ILE-1-α, and tumor necrosis factor, are released. These in turn stimulate the expression of immunomodulating proteins (e.g. HLA-DR) in fibroblasts, thereby perpetuating the autoimmune reaction. Glycosaminoglycans, molecules with considerable hygroscopic properties, significantly contribute to the swelling of orbital tissues (Mann 1995). The concentration of glycosaminoglycans, which are excreted in urine, seems to be an indicator of the activity of the disease (Pappa et al. 1993).

In chronic Graves' disease, muscle fiber damage and continuous proliferation of fibrous tissue leads to fibrosis. At this stage, anti-inflammatory or immunomodulating therapies are no longer effective (Mann 1995).

Psychosomatic Aspects

Increasingly – and judging from our experience with more than 800 patients rightly so – attention is being focused on the role of psychosomatic factors in the onset as well as in the clinical course of Graves' disease. Often an experience of loss (such as the death of someone close, loss of one's job, divorce, or a house move resulting in the loss of one's social network) or long-term physical and emotional stress can trigger or worsen the disease.

Therefore, every patient with suspected Graves' disease should be evaluated with regard to his or her present personal situation (Bacci and Giammarco 1993; Rosch 1993).

Clinical Picture and Patterns of CT Findings

Clinically, Graves' disease is characterized by progressive proptosis with lid retraction, chemosis, and hyperemia above the extraocular muscle insertions at the globe, the typical symptoms being burning and hyperlacrimation and a sensation of pressure behind the globe. Slowly progressive unilateral or asymmetrical forms of the disease may be mistaken for an orbital tumor, particularly if a myasthenic component, present in up to 5% of patients, leads to ptosis instead of lid retraction. Massive swelling or fibrosis may result in restricted ocular motility with double vision. In extreme cases, the optic nerve or its vascular supply may be compressed within the orbital apex by the swollen muscles or by the orbital fat due to an acute increase in volume caused by water retention. Surgical decompression may then become necessary.

Attempts to group signs and symptoms in order to assign a patient to a certain "grade" of Graves' disease, to enable doctors to better quantify therapeutic success, have produced various classifications. The best-known and, with adaptations, the most widely used classification is the Werner classification. As Boergen and Pickhardt explained in 1991, this classification suggests that ocular symptoms should follow a particular course from grade I to VI, which, in fact, they do not. This classification encourages confusion of direct and indirect signs, such as exposure keratopathy and proptosis: the latter being an indirect sign, the degree of which depends on the form of the orbit, the amount of inflammatory infiltration, the water content of the orbital fat, the size of the globes, etc. Classifications also promote confusion of primary signs and symptoms and their sequelae. Visual loss, for example, may have numerous causes: surface irritation as a result of proptosis; deformation of the globe causing irregular astigmatism as a result of compression by enlarged extraocular muscles; or optic nerve compression. Restriction of ocular motility and diplopia, for example, often develop not before the transformation of muscle into fibrous tissue, after the original inflammatory process is long burnt out.

Because of these inaccuracies, the use of classifications has probably done more to obscure than to clarify the results of therapeutic studies. Proptosis and limitation of eye movements should be documented photographically and with the help of standardized motility tests. Functional tests should be supplemented with objective measurements performed by an experienced ophthalmologist. Standardized criteria of documentation are a prerequisite for comparing the effectiveness of different therapeutic measures.

Polymyositic Form of Graves' Disease

The polymyositic form of Graves' disease with several extraocular muscles of both orbits affected, is the most common form of Graves' disease. In some cases extreme enlargement of the proximal parts, which converge in the orbital apex, can lead to optic nerve compression (Cases 35, 38). Exact visualization is best achieved with CT reformations along their course and/or at an angle of about 90° to their course. Exact visualization confirms the diagnosis and usually also offers explanations for functional deficits. Ocular motility is frequently restricted more by impaired relaxation than by impaired contraction, so the main restriction is in the direction opposite to the muscle's primary function. Longstanding infiltration causes the replacement of destroyed muscle tissue by fibrous tissue. Collagen fibers within the fibrous tissue undergo shrinkage, which eventually results in a shortening of the extraocular muscle (Case 37). This explains why, in patients with Graves' disease, the globes are often fixed in a downward and inward position. Scar tissue can be visualized by CT and MRI; it appears as a hypodense area or an area of low signal intensity, respectively, within the muscle. In cases of extreme fibrosis the extraocular muscles appear as short, hypodense bands. Visualization of fibrotic changes is helpful for planning the extent of extraocular muscle surgery. In the case of optic nerve dysfunction, CT or MRI visualization is also needed to decide whether or not surgical decompression is indicated. Thin-section CT also shows the signs of long-term increase in intraorbital pressure: impressions of the ethmoidal air cells ("Coca-Cola bottle sign") and erosions of the lateral orbital floor or of the orbital roof due to spontaneous decompression (Cases 32, 34, 35, 38).

R. G., 44-year-old woman

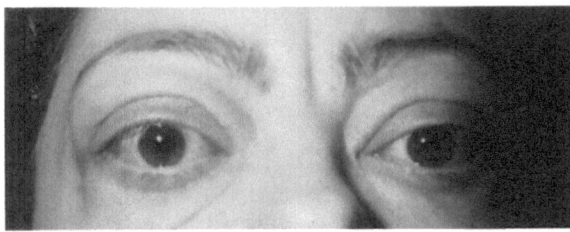

35.1

History and Clinical Findings

Hyperthyroidism diagnosed 11 months ago. For the past 10 months, protrusion of the globe and diplopia.

Near-total thyroidectomy 1 month ago. Since then, worsening of diplopia, visual loss, and reduction of VEP amplitudes indicative of incipient optic nerve compression. Bilaterally, severely restricted ocular motility.

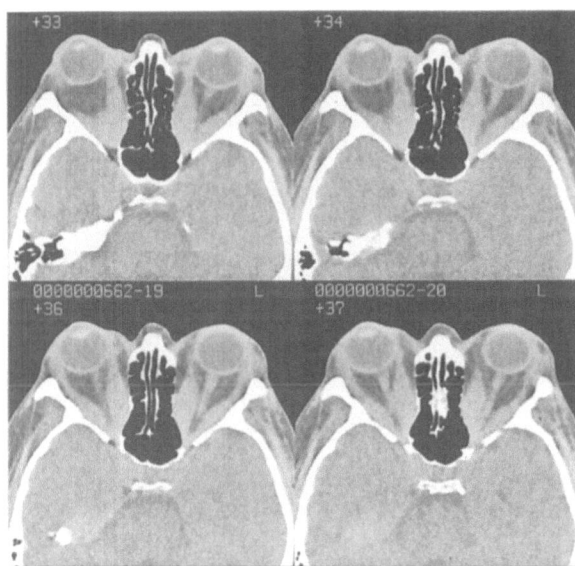

35.2

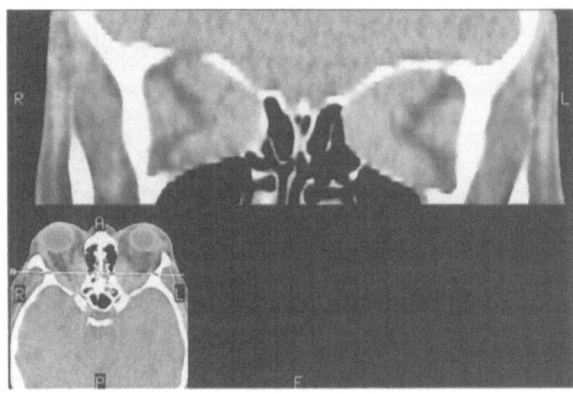

35.3

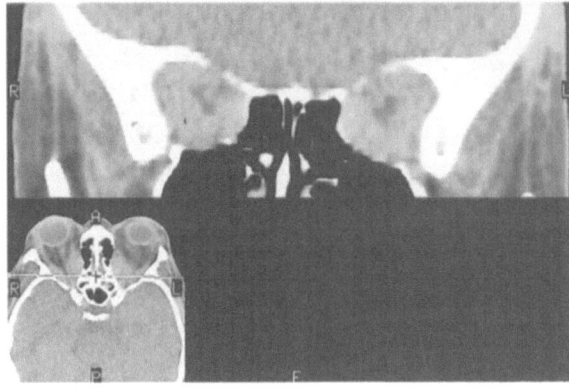

35.4

CT (35.2 – 35.4)

Massive enlargement of extraocular muscles, bilateral impression of the lamina papyracea ("Coca-Cola bottle sign"). Optic nerve compression in the orbital apex. Bilateral exophthalmos. Partial erosions of both orbital roofs, spontaneous decompression.

Diagnosis

Graves' disease, polymyositic form.

Clinical Course

Irradiation of the orbital apex. Four months later, recurrence of clinical signs and symptoms (35.5, 35.6).

(Continued on p. 60)

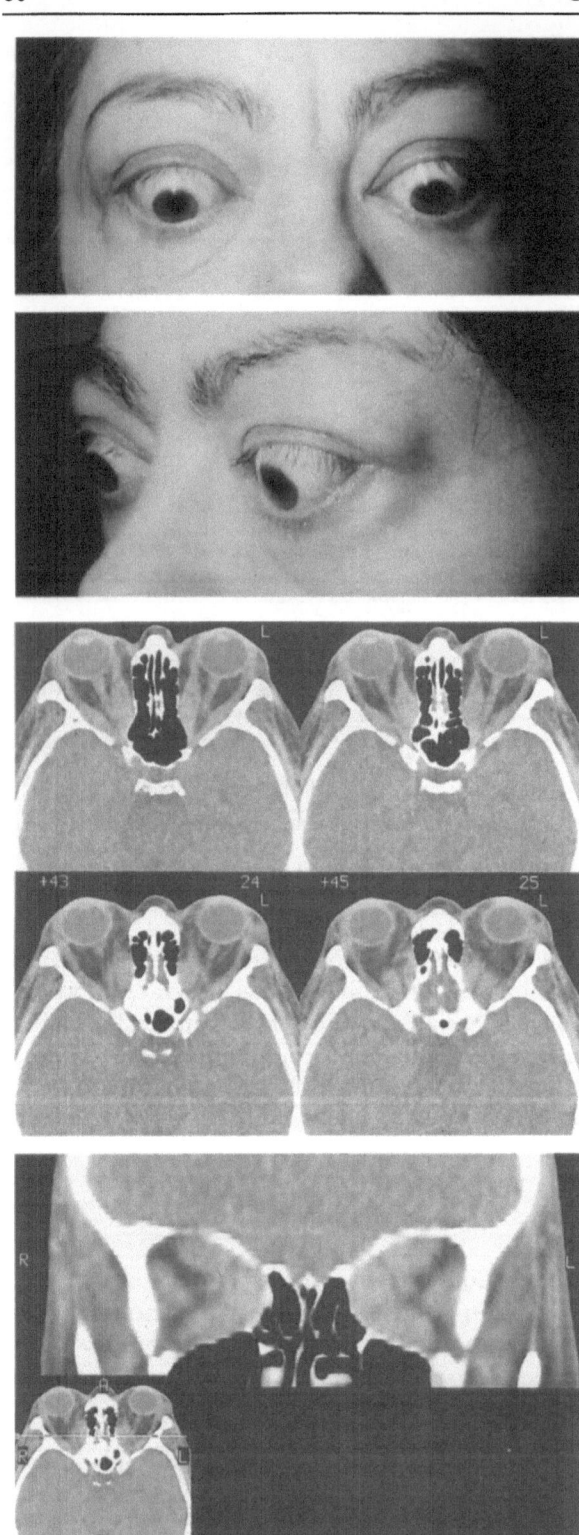

35.5

35.6

35.7

35.8

CT (35.7, 35.8)
No radiographic changes after irradiation of the
orbital apex.

B.B., 52-year-old woman

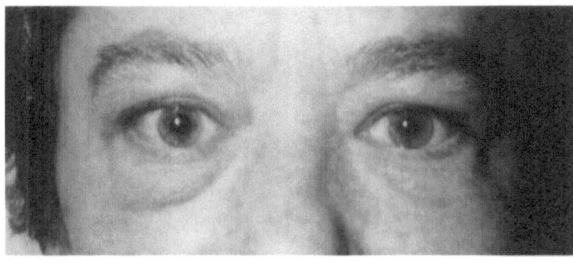

36.1

History and Clinical Findings
Thyroid disorder diagnosed 30 years ago. Hyper-thyroid episode 7 months ago. Near-total thyroid-ectomy 4 months ago.

Visual loss in the right eye for 3 months. Diplopia on right gaze, slight proptosis.

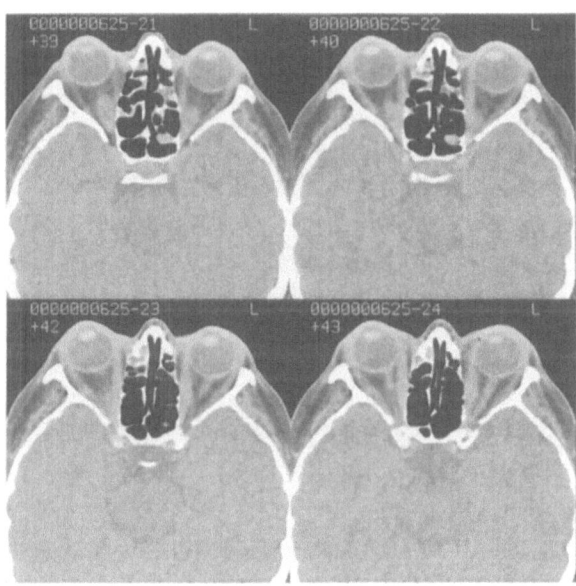

36.2

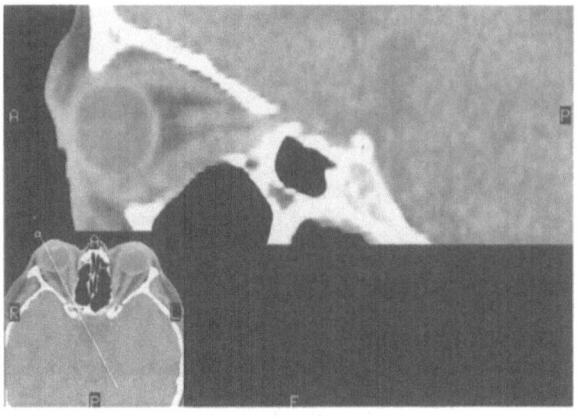

36.3

36.4

CT
Enlargement of most extraocular muscles in both orbits.

Diagnosis
Bilateral Graves' disease, polymyositic form.

G. K., 46-year-old man

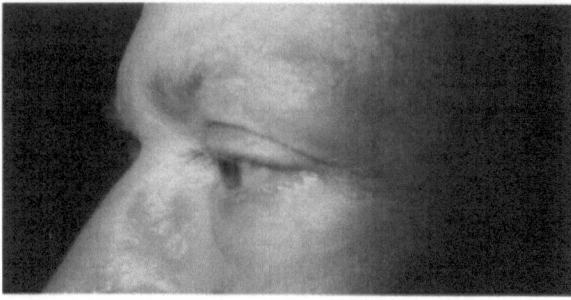

37.1

History and Clinical Findings
Hyperthyroidism diagnosed 4 years ago. Antithyroid medication, presently euthyroid. Progressive bilateral limitation of upward gaze with diplopia.

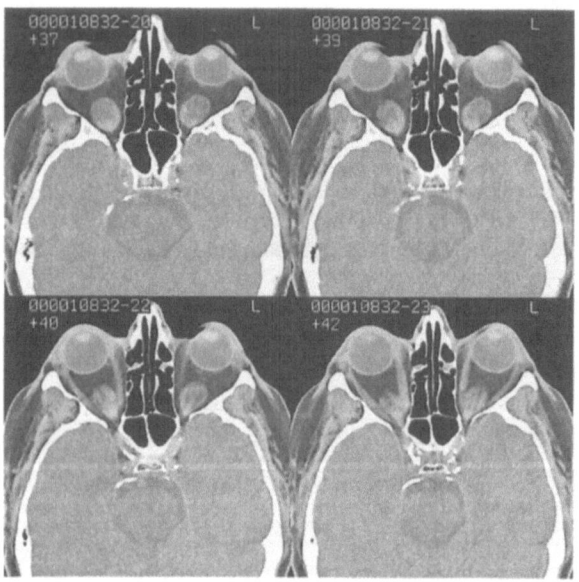

37.2

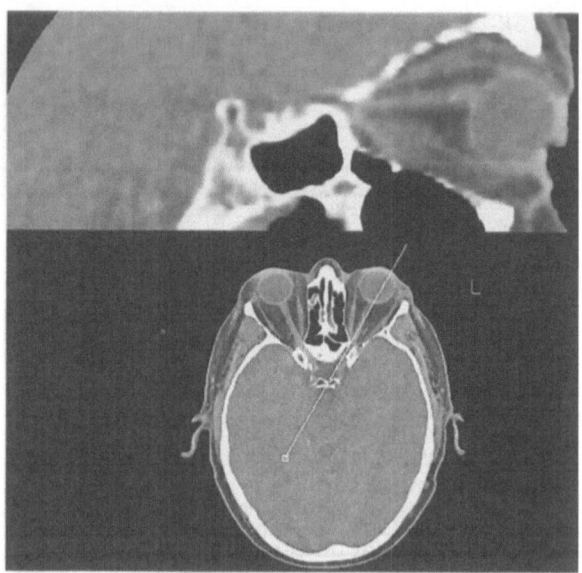

37.3

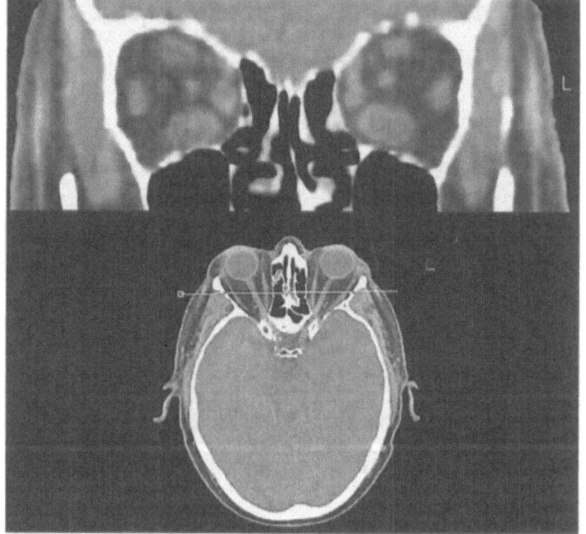

37.4

CT
Enlargement of most extraocular muscles in both orbits, particularly of both inferior rectus muscles, with hypodense areas. Increase in the volume of the orbital fat. Proptosis is slight due to relatively large bony orbits.

Diagnosis
Graves' disease, polymyositic form with fibrotic changes.

Comment
Limitation of upward gaze is caused by the enlargement and fibrosis of the inferior rectus muscles, which cannot fully extend to permit the intended upward gaze.

G. O., 56-year-old woman

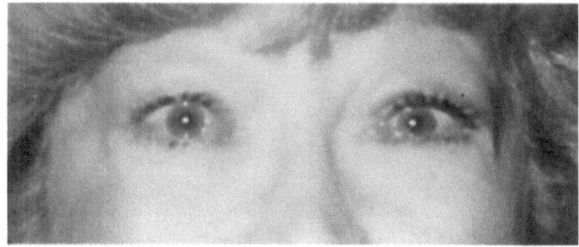

38.1

History and Clinical Findings
Swelling of both upper lids and hyperthyroidism
for the past 12 months.

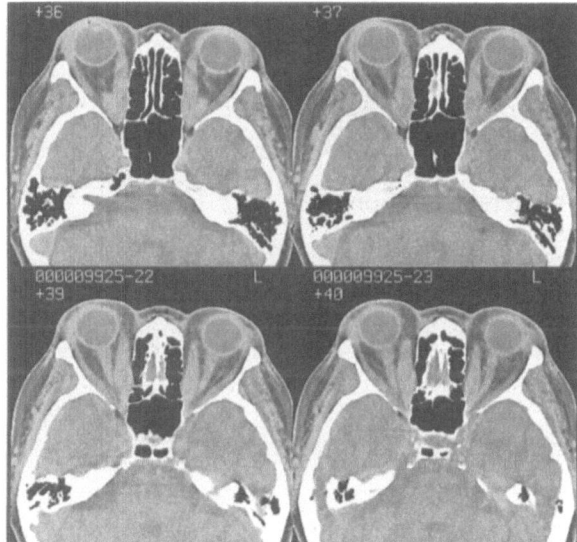

8.2

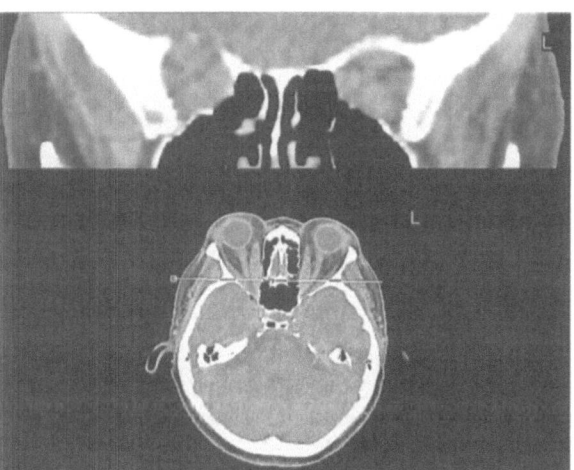

8.3

CT
Severe enlargement of most extraocular muscles,
more prominent in the right orbit. Bilaterally,
increase in the volume of the orbital fat. Focal
excavation of the right orbital roof; the bone is
markedly reduced and partially eroded.

Diagnosis
Bilateral Graves' disease, polymyositic form, optic
nerve compression in the orbital apex, more pronounced in the right orbit. Partial spontaneous
decompression of the right orbital roof.

Clinical Course
After irradiation of the orbital apex, regression
of optic nerve compression and restriction of ocular motility, as well as remission of inflammatory
signs and symptoms.

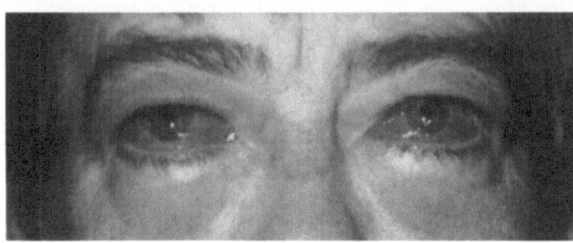

39.1

Patient with thyrotoxicosis and hyperacute onset
of severe ophthalmopathy before and after lateral
decompression.

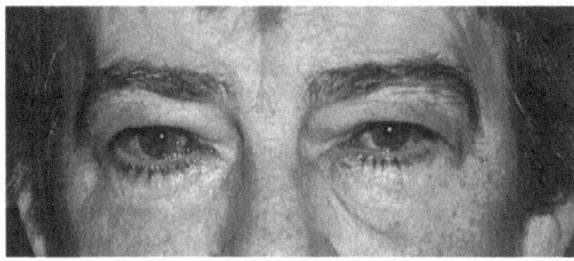

39.2

Before surgical intervention, bilateral reduction of
visual acuity to hand movements. Vision after
decompression was 60/100 on the right and 80/100
on the left.

M. S., 41-year-old woman

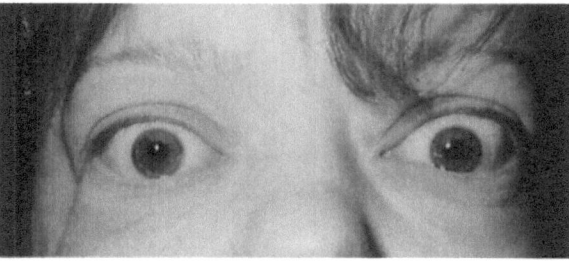

40.1

History and Clinical Findings
Graves' disease with extreme proptosis. Irradiation of the optical apex had been ineffective; surgical decompression on the right side 3 years ago.

Postoperative remission of proptosis of the right eye.

At present bilateral proptosis, more prominent on the left side, and severe lid retraction.

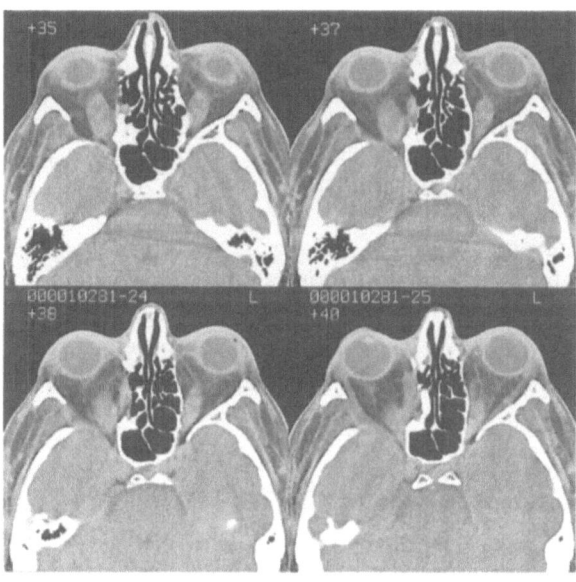

40.2

CT
After removal of the right greater wing of the sphenoid bone and the lamina papyracea, displacement of the extraocular muscles. Due to medial and lateral surgical decompression, proptosis is less prominent on the right side.

Diagnosis
Bilateral polymyositic form of Graves' disease.

Comment
The small size of the bony orbits determines the pronounced proptosis in the presence of only slight enlargement of the extraocular muscles and moderate increase in the volume of the orbital fat.

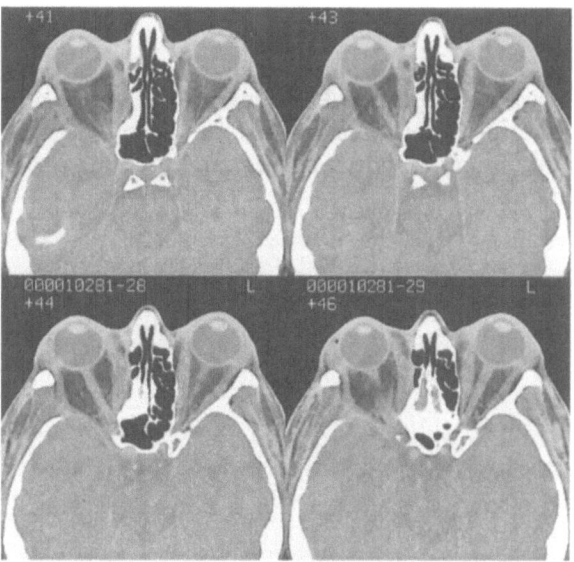

40.3

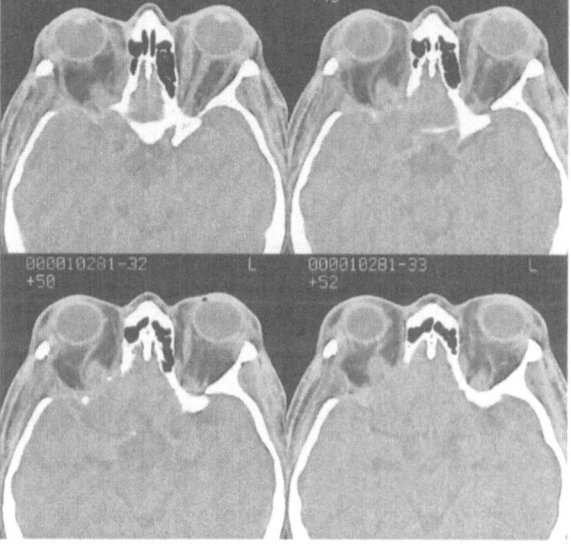

40.4

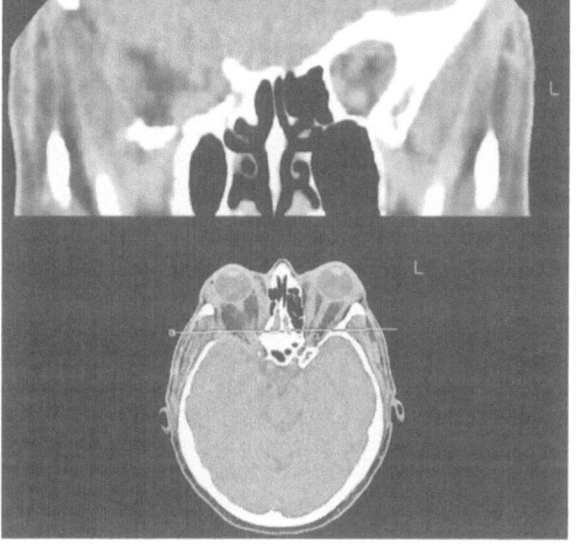

40.5

S.R., 50-year-old woman

History and Clinical Findings
Bilateral proptosis, more prominent on the right side. Bilateral optic nerve compression, papilledema.

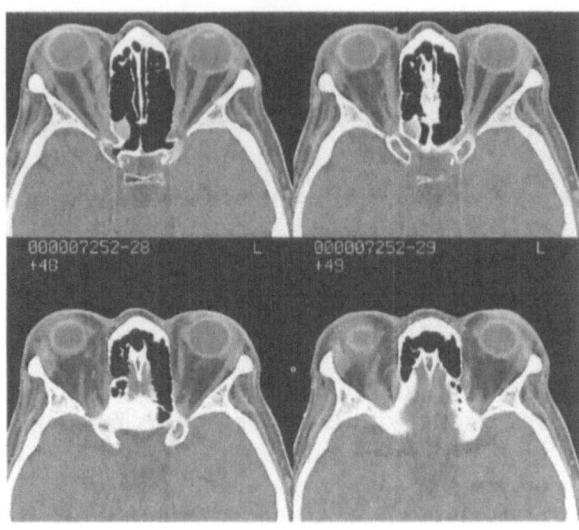

41.2

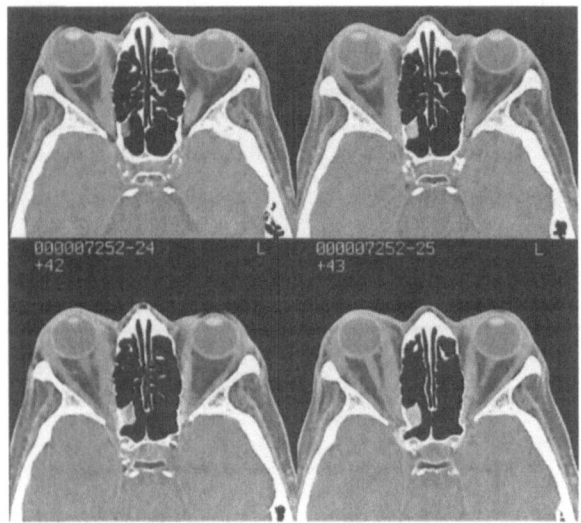

41.1

CT (41.1, 41.2)
Extraocular muscle enlargement, more pronounced on the right side. Moderate bilateral increase in the volume of the orbital fat. Bilateral proptosis and lacrimal gland enlargement.

Diagnosis
Polymyositic type of Graves' disease, more pronounced on the right side.

Therapy
Lateral surgical decompression of both orbits.

(Continued on p. 67)

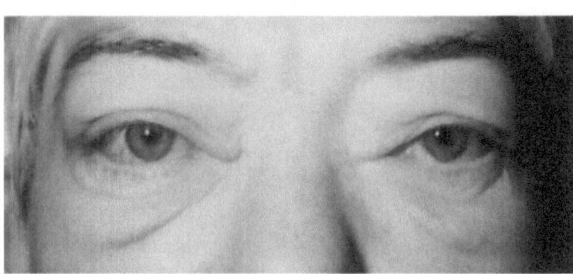

41.3

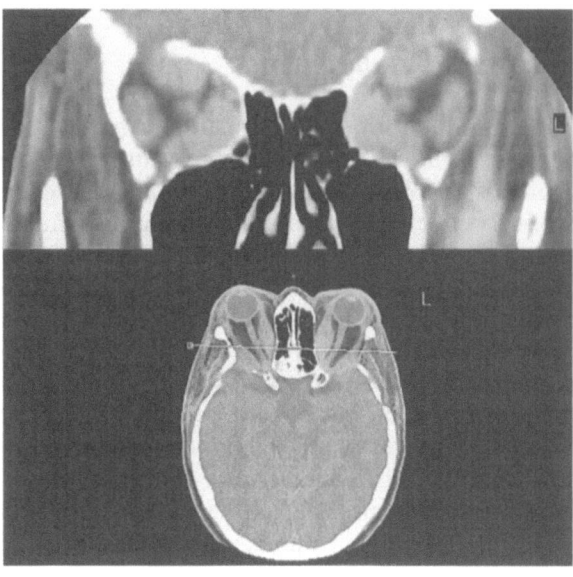

41.6

CT (41.4–41.6)

One year after lateral surgical decompression. Parts of both greater wings of the sphenoid bone and both orbital roofs have been removed. Bilateral concave impression of the lamina papyracea ("Coca-Cola bottle sign"). Compared to the previous CT scans, noticeable increase in extraocular muscle enlargement.

Comment

Proptosis is unchanged despite extensive surgical decompression. This is due to the considerable increase in muscle enlargement which without decompression would have caused further increase in exophthalmos.

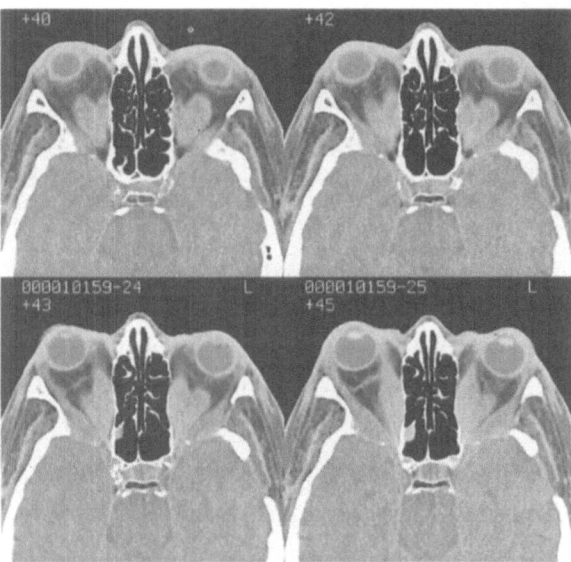

41.4

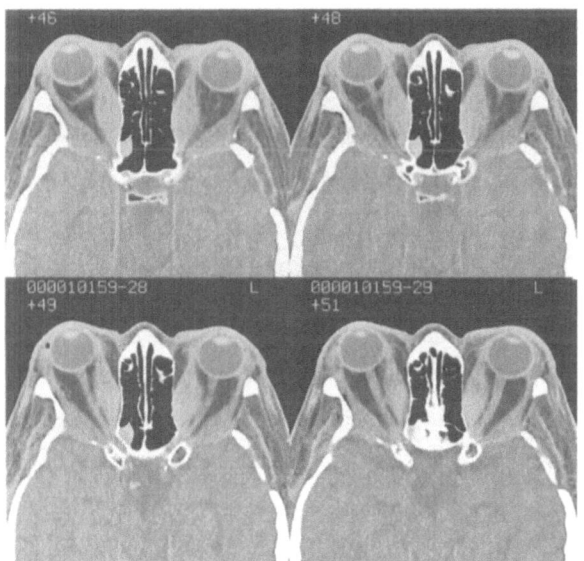

41.5

Mono- or Paucimyositic Form of Graves' Disease

In the mono- or the paucimyositic form of Graves' disease, usually only one or two muscles of one orbit are affected. The inferior rectus muscle is more frequently affected than is the upper muscle complex. This form usually takes a slowly progressive course. Symptoms such as restricted eye movements or double vision may develop over a period of several years. When symptoms occur, the previous thyroid disease may not be remembered. If the affected muscle is sectioned obliquely in CT or MRI, it appears as an oval hyperdense structure and may be misdiagnosed as a tumor of the orbital apex. This may lead to unnecessary surgery and cause irreversible damage (Brismar et al. 1976; Unsöld 1989). If only one inferior rectus muscle is involved, surgical correction of the muscle is frequently all that is needed to restore ocular motility. Whether and to what extent the different forms of Graves' disease correlate with certain immunological constellations remains to be investigated.

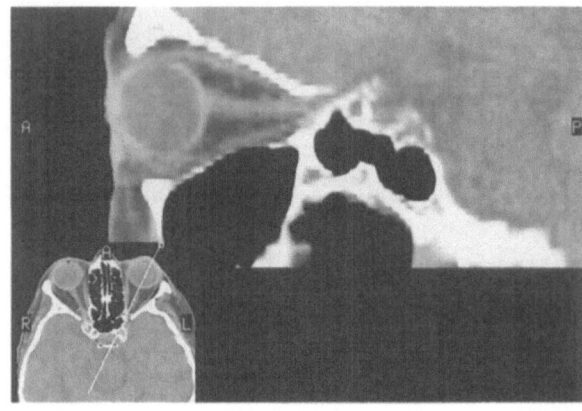

42.2

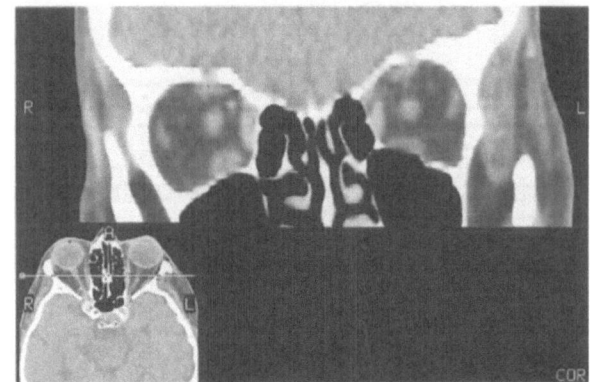

42.3

S. L., 70-year-old woman

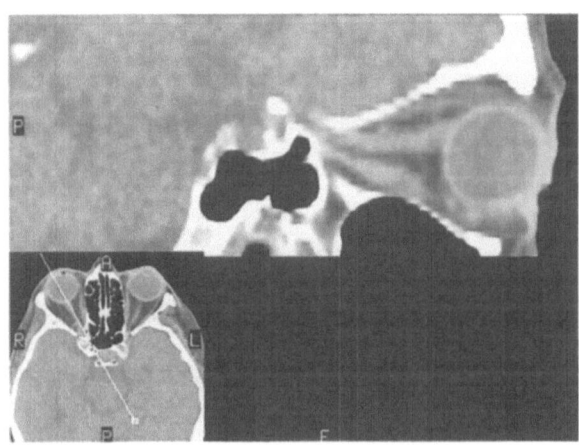

42.1

42.4

CT
Unilateral spindle-shaped enlargement of the right inferior rectus muscle.

Diagnosis
Graves' disease, monomyositic form, unilateral.

Comment
Because of low visual acuity the patient did not perceive double vision until after cataract surgery. Double vision is caused by the enlarged, immobile inferior rectus muscle.

History and Clinical Findings
Cataract extraction on the right eye 6 months ago. Since then limitation of upward gaze in the right eye and diplopia.

N. J., 45-year-old woman

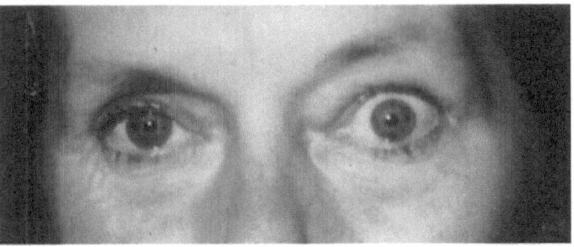

43.1

History and Clinical Findings
Progressive retraction of the left upper lid.

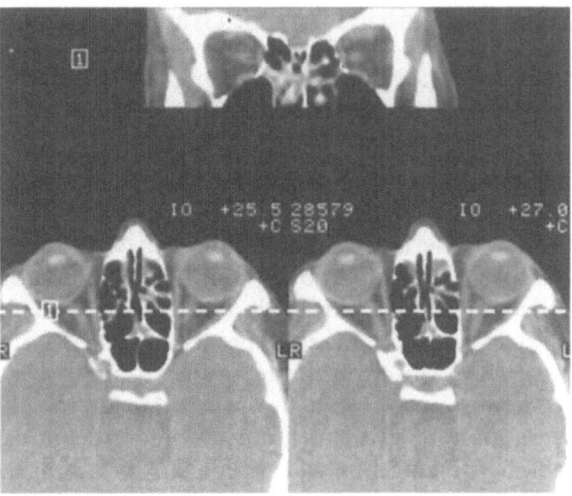

43.4

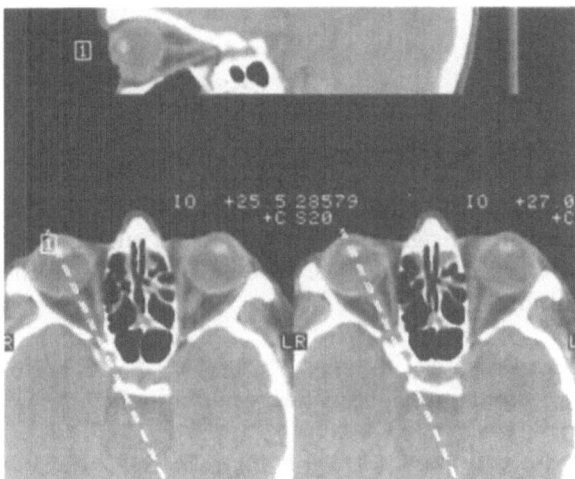

43.2

CT
Enlargement of the left upper eye muscle complex and decrease of the upper extraconal orbital fat.

Diagnosis
Unilateral Graves' disease, monomyositic form.

Clinical Course
Hyperthyroidism was confirmed by laboratory assessment.

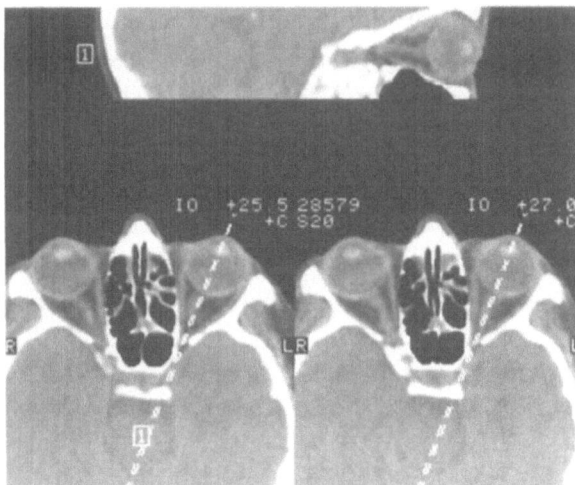

43.3

Dacryoadenitic Form of Graves' disease

In the dacryoadenitic form of Graves' disease, it is initially only the lacrimal gland that is infiltrated with no concomitant changes in the extraocular muscles or the orbital fat (Case 44). Sometimes a slight secondary enlargement of the levator palpebrae muscle and lid retraction can be observed (Case 6). This is probably due to inflammatory cells migrating from the lacrimal gland into the levator palpebrae muscle, the distal part of which is situated closely underneath the lacrimal gland. Infiltration may result in fibrosis and thereby lid retraction. At this stage, muscle enlargement can usually no longer be visualized.

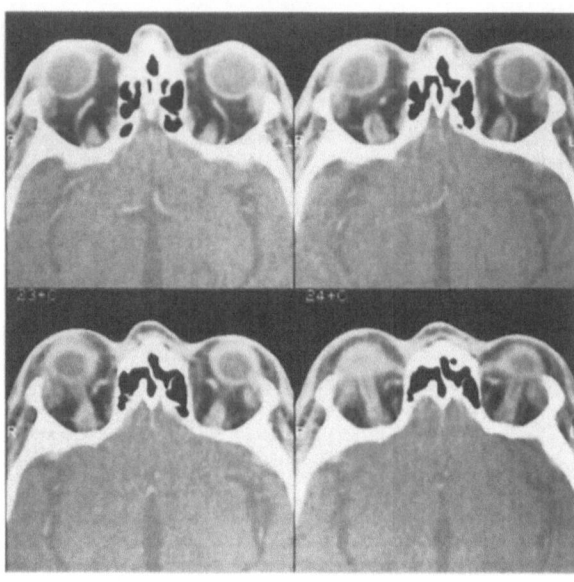

44.2

CT
Enlargement of both lacrimal glands, more prominent on the right side. No significant enlargement of extraocular muscles. Moderate increase in the volume of the orbital fat.

Diagnosis
Graves' disease, mainly dacryoadenitic form.

Histopathology *(lacrimal gland)*
Moderate chronic dacryoadenitis, accentuation of inflammatory infiltration around the lacrimal ducts.

B. H.-P., 47-year-old man

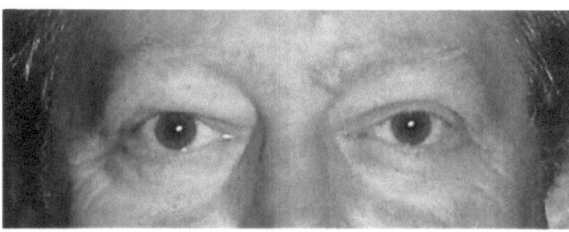

44.1

History and Clinical Findings
Hyperlacrimation and slight proptosis for the past 5 months. Hyperthyroidism was confirmed, as were thyroid-related antibodies. Bilateral proptosis, more prominent on the left side for 3 months. Moderate retraction of both upper lids.

Presentation because of further increase in proptosis.

Increase in Volume of Orbital Fat in Graves' Disease

Increase in the volume of the orbital fat in Graves' disease is caused by the accumulation of fluid by hygroscopic substances (glycosaminoglycans) within the orbital fat in the presence of impaired barrier function of the orbital vessels.

One may easily fail to diagnose this form of Graves' disease, particularly in less severe cases, as there is considerable interindividual variation in the volume of the orbital fat. Evidence for an increase in the volume of the orbital fat is provided by an enlargement of the intraconal and extraconal fat space and the forward displacement of the lacrimal glands. Rarely does this form of Graves' disease lead to a considerable increase in intraorbital pressure or optic nerve compression. At this time the extraocular muscles may be normal in size. In some cases, muscles may become infiltrated months or even years later. Since the increase in the volume of the orbital fat is caused by hygroscopic substances rather than by inflammatory infiltration, radiation is not a promising therapeutic option.

Differential Diagnosis

The *polymyositic form* of Graves' disease is to be distinguished from muscle enlargement or infiltration of different origin, as in systemic lymphomas, subacute inflammatory orbital pseudotumor, multiple metastases, and orbital involvement in somatotropin-producing pituitary neoplasms (Case 45) (Dal Pozzo and Boschi 1982). Whether or not diffuse enlargement of extraocular muscles in lymphoproliferative disease or in carcinomas is a paraneoplastic phenomenon is not clear and remains to be investigated.

Slight enlargement of several extraocular muscles can also be observed in cavernous sinus fistulas, which, however, are mostly unilateral. Muscle enlargement tends to affect the proximal parts only (Merlis et al. 1982). In addition, cavernous sinus fistulas cause dilatation of the superior ophthalmic vein continuing anteriorly and superiorly into the supratrochlear vein (Cases 18, 102) and considerable episcleral venous injection.

Metastases cause focal enlargement of the extraocular muscles, which can only be mistaken for Graves' disease at the very beginning.

The *monomyositic form* of Graves' disease must be distinguished from ocular myositis in inflammatory orbital pseudotumor, whereby the latter may be recognized from its acute and painful clinical course and from marked involvement of the tendon. Unilateral muscle enlargement can also be observed in tumors primarily arising within the extraocular muscles, such as granular cell tumors, rhabdomyosarcomas, fibromas or hematomas.

There are numerous differential diagnoses to the *dacryoadenitic form* of Graves' disease, as it cannot be distinguished by radiological means from other infiltrations of the lacrimal gland, for instance in viral disease, sarcoidosis, inflammatory systemic disease, lymphoma or other forms of leukemia. Whenever the association of lacrimal gland enlargement with thyroid disease is not unequivocal, particularly if enlargement is bilateral, a surgical biopsy should be performed in order not to miss an early stage of systemic inflammatory or neoplastic disease. Biopsy of suspected mixed tumors of the lacrimal gland must never be performed. If a mixed tumor cannot be ruled out with safety by thin-section CT and MRI, primary en-bloc resection of the lesion should be performed, because of the dramatic increase in the rate of recurrence and mortality after biopsy or partial resection.

Every patient with diffuse uni- or bilateral lacrimal gland enlargement needs a thorough medical examination.

F.H., 56-year-old woman

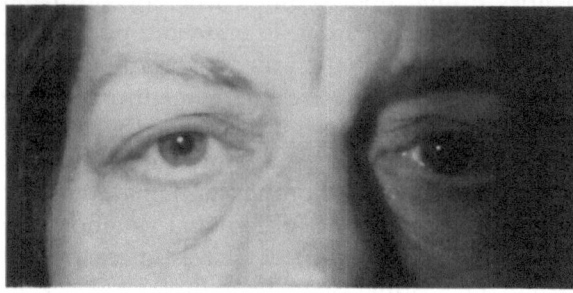

45.1

History and Clinical Findings

Binasal visual field defects, destruction of VEP amplitudes, acromegalic appearance. Known adenoma of the pituitary gland with hypersecretion of somatotropin and prolactin. Other pituitary axes normal. T_3, T_4, and thyroid-related antibodies normal.

MRI (not shown)

Extended intrasellar adenoma of the pituitary gland, not affecting the anterior visual pathway.
    Therapy with bromocriptine was initiated.

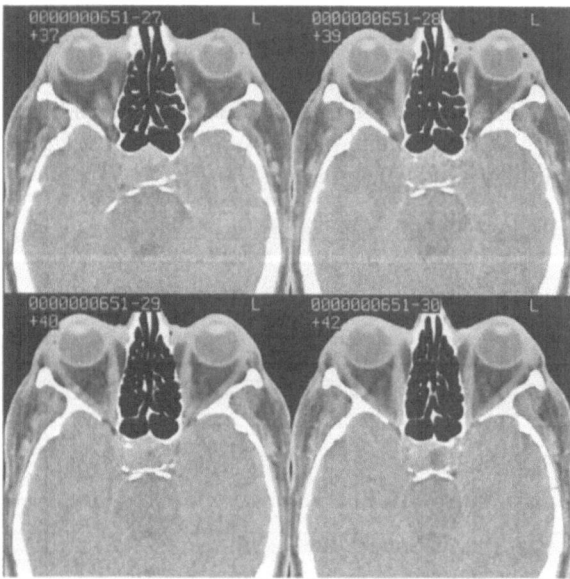

45.2

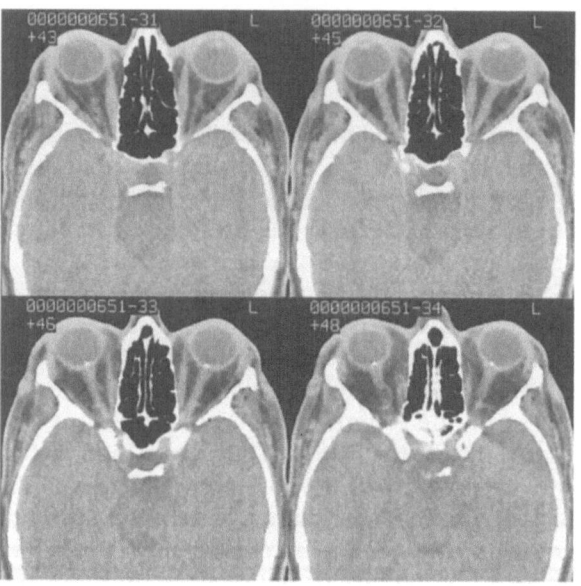

45.3

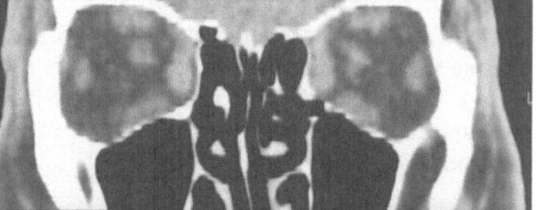

45.4

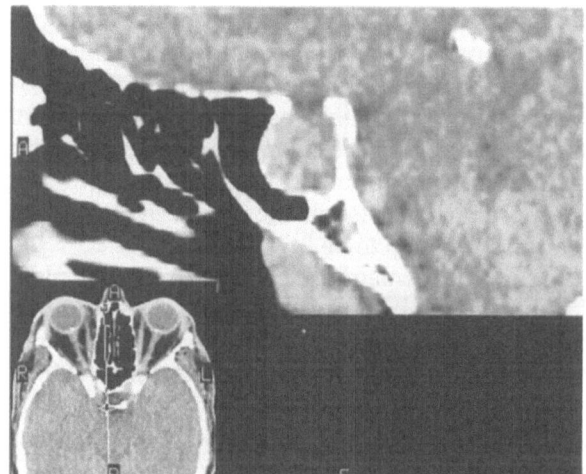

45.5

(Continued on p. 73)

CT

Bilateral drusen of the optic nerve head (these can not be visualized on MRI). Slight proptosis and symmetrical enlargement of the extraocular muscles, slight enlargement of both lacrimal glands. Extended intrasellar adenoma of the pituitary gland with marked ballooning of the sella.

Comment

Enlargement of extraocular muscles and of the lacrimal glands are occasionally observed in somatotropin-secreting tumors, particularly adenomas (Dal Pozzo and Boschi 1982).

The binasal scotomas are caused by drusen of the optic disc, which cannot be visualized by MRI.

4 Inflammatory Orbital Pseudotumor

Definition and Etiology

"Birch-Hirschfeld (1905) is usually credited with defining the existence of a pseudotumor group of diseases. His classification included three types: (1) orbital tumor which subsides spontaneously, (2) exophthalmos which at operation had no distinct tumefaction causing it and which microscopically displays chronic inflammatory tissue, and (3) exophthalmos which at operation is caused by an abnormal orbital mass which has been created by a nonspecific inflammatory reaction."

(Jakobiec and Jones 1978)

Later, particularly prior to the development of CT, the term was used for a variety of different orbital lesions now defined as distinct disease entities, such as foreign body reactions, inflammations within orbital capillary hemangiomas, dermoid cysts, etc. Essential qualifications were provided by Blodi and Gass (1968) and particularly by Jakobiec and Jones (1978), who defined inflammatory orbital pseudotumor as an "unspecific inflammation of orbital structures in the absence of systemic or local disease". This definition must be further qualified since certain forms of inflammatory orbital pseudotumor, in particular ocular myositis and soft-tissue masses, may well be associated with proven systemic inflammatory disease, such as soft-tissue masses in panarteritis nodosa or Wegener's granulomatosis, ocular myositis in rheumatoid arthritis or paraneoplastic syndromes.

Inflammatory orbital pseudotumor is characterized by acute, usually unilateral, severe periorbital inflammation and pain. Inflammatory orbital pseudotumor rarely occurs bilaterally. In some cases the onset may be subacute. Therefore, the clinical spectrum of inflammatory orbital pseudotumor is rather wide as is reflected by the variety of different CT findings. The most characteristic symptom of all forms of inflammatory orbital pseudotumor is intense pain, extending beyond the orbit and frequently developing into a migraine-like hemicrania.

It was not until the development of thin-section CT that diagnosis and differential diagnosis of the different forms of inflammatory orbital pseudotumor became possible with a high degree of safety.

With regard to etiology the clinical association of inflammatory orbital pseudotumor with auto-immune disease as well as the histological finding of infiltration by immune cells indicate an immunopathogenetic mechanism. This assumption is further substantiated by the rapid response to, and the frequently definitive cure by, steroid treatment.

Inflammatory orbital pseudotumor can affect every orbital structure. The different forms of inflammatory orbital pseudotumor may be distinguished by different patterns of CT findings, necessary for differential diagnosis. Marked involvement of the muscle tendon in ocular myositis is most helpful in differentiating ocular myositis from other pathological lesions causing muscle enlargement (p. 173, Plate 15a). The diffusely infiltrating form of inflammatory orbital pseudotumor is to be differentiated from other orbital infiltrations (p. 177, Plate 16a). With regard to therapy, it is crucial to distinguish the different forms of inflammatory orbital pseudotumor from lesions which appear similar with regard to the patterns of CT-findings, but are of different etiology.

Clinical Picture and CT-Patterns

Ocular Myositis-Tendonitis

Ocular myositis-tendonitis is the most common form of inflammatory orbital pseudotumor. Usually, considerable enlargement of one extraocular muscle and its tendon can be visualized. Only rarely is more than one muscle affected. This form of inflammatory orbital pseudotumor is accompanied by restricted ocular motility and double vision, increasing pain with eye movements, considerable periorbital swelling, hyperemia above the muscle insertion, proptosis, and chemosis. The onset of symptoms is generally hyperacute.

The characteristic CT and MRI finding is enlargement of one extraocular muscle with severe swelling of the muscle tendon, particularly at its insertion. Further typical findings include concomitant inflammatory reaction of the adjacent Tenon's capsule and the lacrimal gland, as well as severe inflammation of the lids, which may be mistaken for orbital cellulitis (Cases 13, 14).

Basically, all extraocular muscles may be affected. Most frequently affected are the medial and lateral rectus muscles. If the lateral rectus muscle or the upper muscle complex is affected there is often accompanying swelling of the lacrimal gland. Myositis-tendonitis of the inferior oblique muscle, the insertion of which is situated below the posterior pole of the globe, can, due to concomitant inflammation of the Tenon's capsule and adjacent tissues, lead to choroidal folds and subsequent visual loss. This may, together with the disturbances of ocular motility, imitate an orbital apex syndrome.

Distinct involvement of the tendon is an important diagnostic criterion for distinguishing ocular myositis from the monomyositic form of Graves' disease (Case 13). In Graves' disease only muscle tissue is affected. Ocular myositis may also be part of a paraneoplastic syndrome in patients with certain carcinomas (mainly those of the breast, the lung, and the prostate). Neoplastic infiltration of a muscle is usually not painful and never involves the tendon. Sparing of the tendon also helps to differentiate posttraumatic intramuscular hematoma from ocular myositis. Primary tumors within extraocular muscles, such as granular-cell tumor, rhabdomyosarcoma, and solitary fibroma, are rare and generally not painful.

A peculiar form of myositis-tendonitis affects the superior oblique muscle and/or its tendon (Case 50). It causes acute-onset vertical diplopia because the enlarged tendon cannot move freely within the trochlea. The clinical picture is also known as "Brown's Syndrome" (Stammen et al. 1995).

K.R., 23-year-old woman

History and Clinical Findings
Periorbital pain, swelling and hyperemia 2 weeks ago. Complete remission of signs and symptoms was spontaneous.

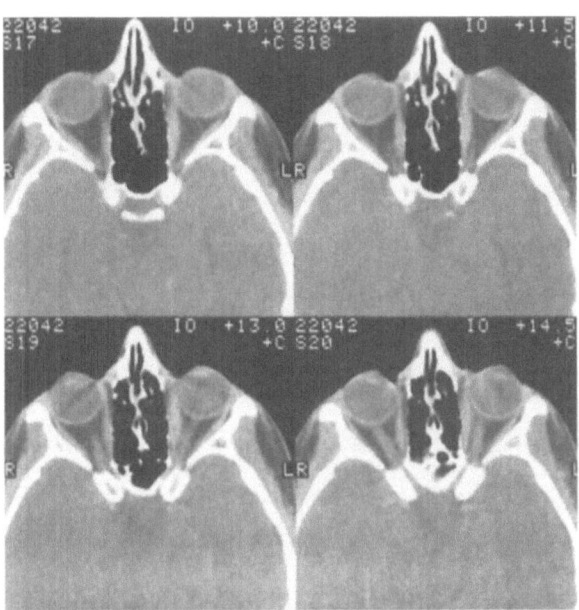

46.1

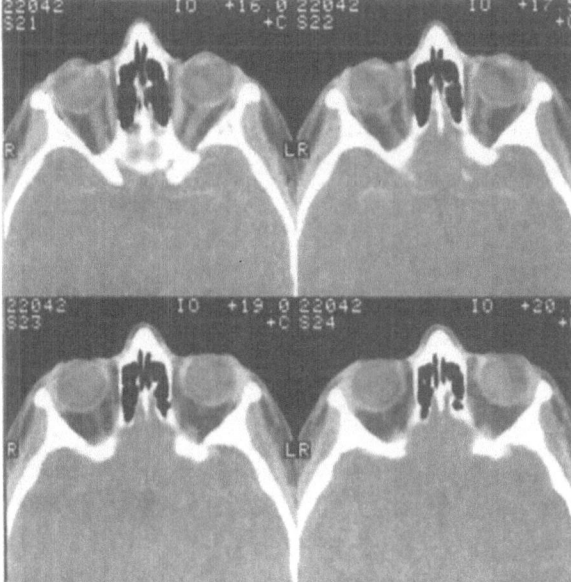

46.2

CT
Enlargement of the left medial rectus muscle and its tendon.

Diagnosis
Myositis-tendonitis of the left medial rectus muscle: myositic form of inflammatory orbital pseudotumor.

K.A., 29-year-old woman

History and Clinical Findings
Pain in the area of the lateral right orbit for 2 weeks. Double vision in left gaze.

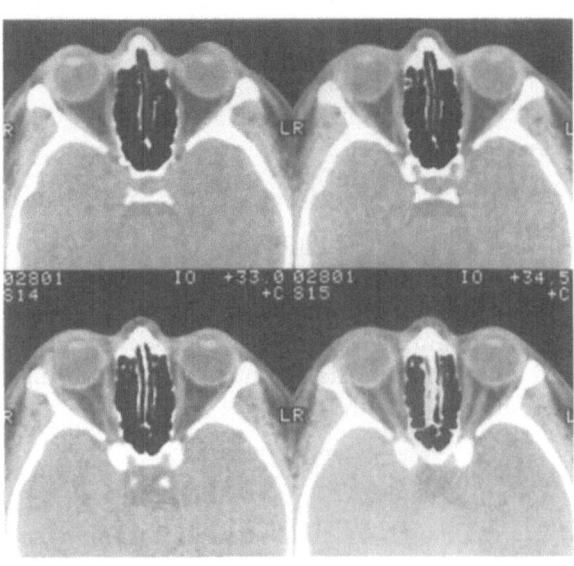

47.1

CT
Slight enlargement of the right lateral rectus muscle and its tendon.

Diagnosis
Myositis-tendonitis of the right lateral rectus muscle: myositic form of inflammatory orbital pseudotumor.

S. H., 60-year-old man

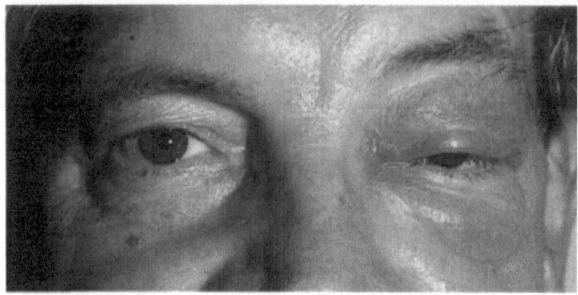

48.1

History and Clinical Findings
Recurrent bouts of rheumatoid arthritis, serologically confirmed, for the past 20 years. One year
ago and again 3 days ago, acute periorbital swelling
and hyperemia, ptosis, chemosis and narrowing of
the palpebral fissure.

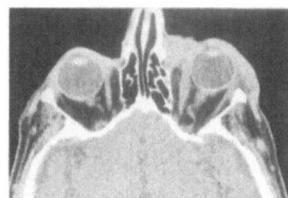

48.2

CT
Enlargement of the medial rectus muscle and massive enlargement of its tendon. Extreme swelling of
the adjacent soft tissue.

Diagnosis
Myositis-tendonitis of the medial rectus muscle:
myositic form of inflammatory orbital pseudotumor.

Clinical Course
Complete remission after several days of steroid
treatment (beginning with 100 mg prednisolone,
gradually reducing the dose).

L. K-H., 44-year-old man

History and Clinical Findings
Stabbing and throbbing periorbital pain in the right eye for the past 3 weeks.

Chemosis and visual loss for 2 weeks. Increasing pain with eye movements and pressure on the globe. Choroidal folds.

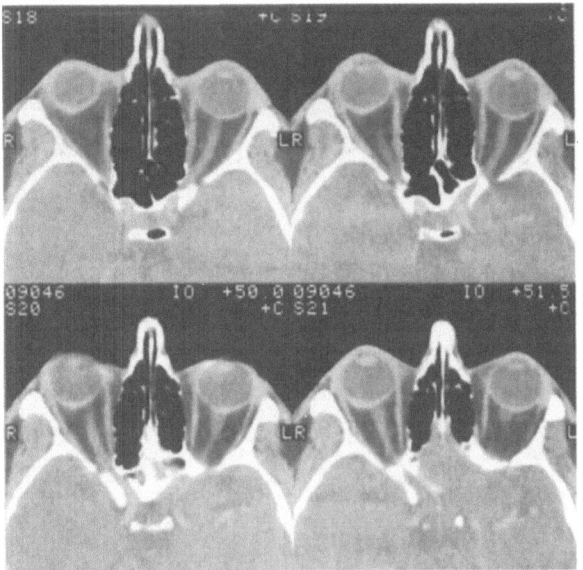

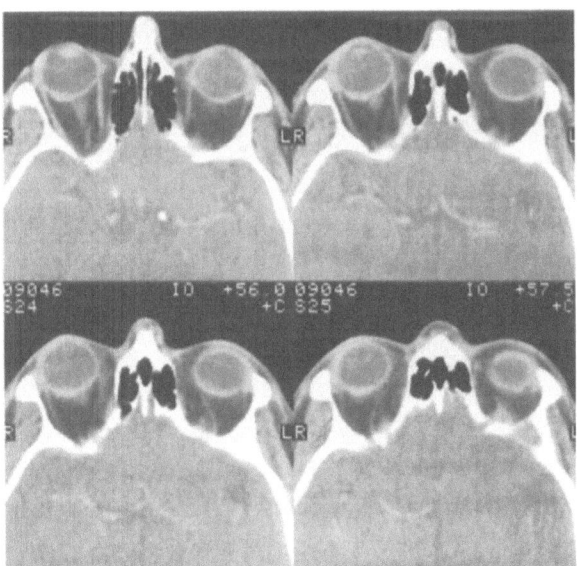

CT
Enlargement of the tendon of the right inferior oblique muscle, mainly at its insertion.

Diagnosis
Myositis-tendonitis of the right inferior oblique muscle: myositic form of inflammatory orbital pseudotumor.

Clinical Course
Systemic steroid therapy (beginning with 100 mg prednisolone, gradually reducing the dose). Complete remission of signs and symptoms within a 3-day period. Decreasing the dose caused recurrence of pain and double vision in upward gaze.

Control CT 2 weeks later: no pathological findings.

49.1

9.2

H. M., 30-year-old man

History and Clinical Findings
Limited upward gaze in the right eye, particularly on adduction, as well as double vision for the past 3 weeks. Sensation of pressure in the right eye.

Brown's syndrome suspected (superior oblique muscle tendon syndrome).

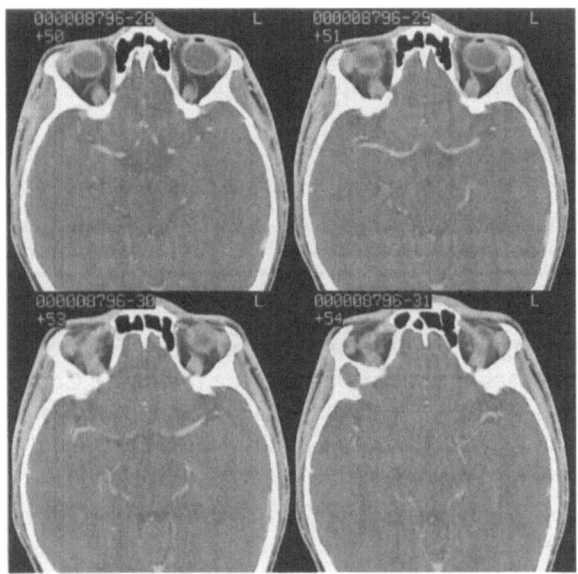

50.1

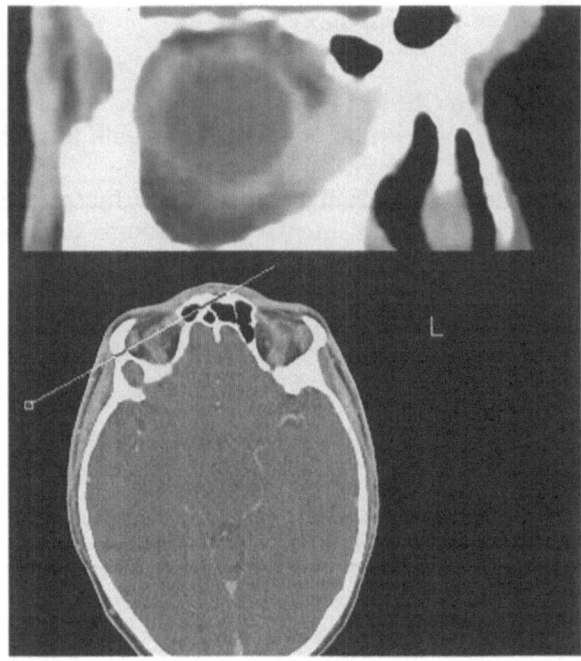

50.2

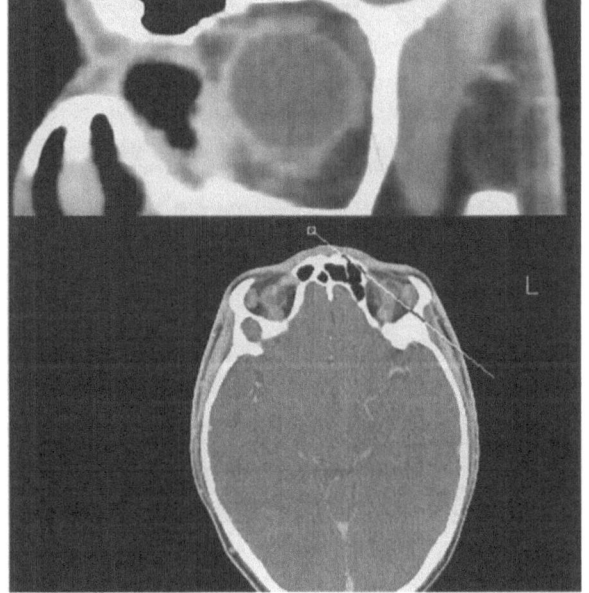

50.3

CT
Enlargement of the tendon of the right superior oblique muscle.

Diagnosis
Brown's syndrome

Comment
The enlarged tendon cannot move freely within the trochlea and vertical eye movements are therefore restricted.

Scleritic-Tenonitic Form
of Inflammatory Orbital Pseudotumor

The scleritic-tenonitic form of inflammatory orbital pseudotumor is characterized by severe pain
around the globe, slight proptosis, and, due to the
involvement of the muscles' insertions, by the
worsening of pain with eye movement. Involvement of the sclera and Tenon's capsule near the
posterior pole may cause choroidal folds. Involvement of the anterior parts of the sclera and Tenon's
capsule near the posterior pole leads to episcleral
and scleral venous injection. Concomitant swelling
of the lacrimal gland can frequently be observed
in scleritis-tenonitis. Acute onset of severe pain is
the chief complaint. The scleritic-tenonitic form of
inflammatory orbital pseudotumor frequently affects patients with systemic inflammatory disease
or malignant tumors. Its diagnosis, particularly
the diagnosis of posterior scleritis, can accurately
be established by thin-section CT with contrast
enhancement: enlargement and infiltration of the
wall of the globe as well as infiltration of Tenon's
capsule can clearly be visualized (Case 53). After
a few days of steroid treatment (beginning with
100 mg prednisolone, gradually reducing the dose),
findings usually subside and can no longer be
visualized.

Because of the association with systemic inflammatory and neoplastic disease, all patients
with the scleritic-tenonitic form of inflammatory
orbital pseudotumor need a complete medical
examination.

B. M., 50-year-old woman

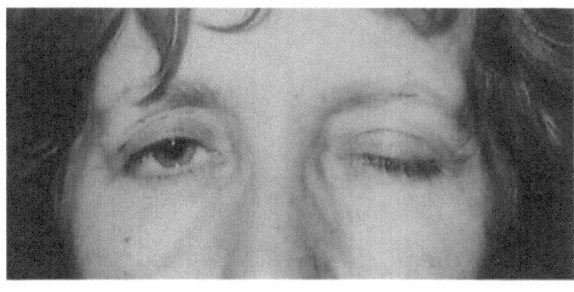

51.1

History and Clinical Findings
Pain in the area of the left eye, ptosis, and left temporal headache.

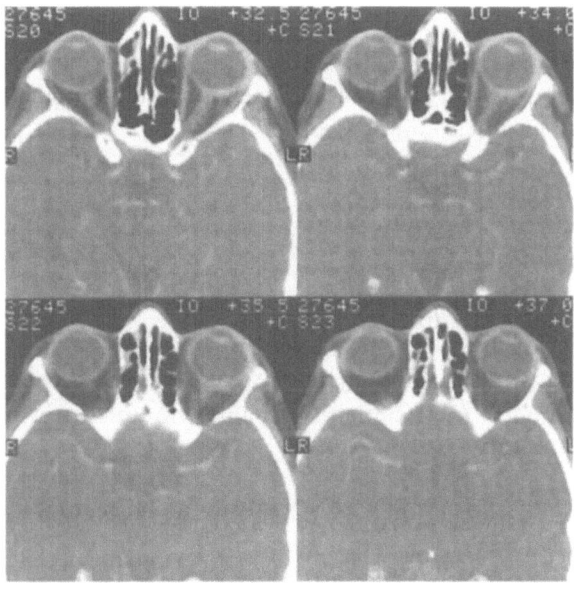

51.2

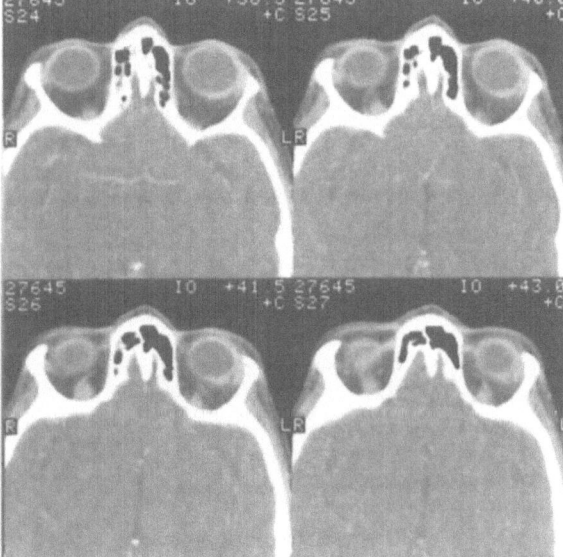

(Continued on p. 82)

51.3

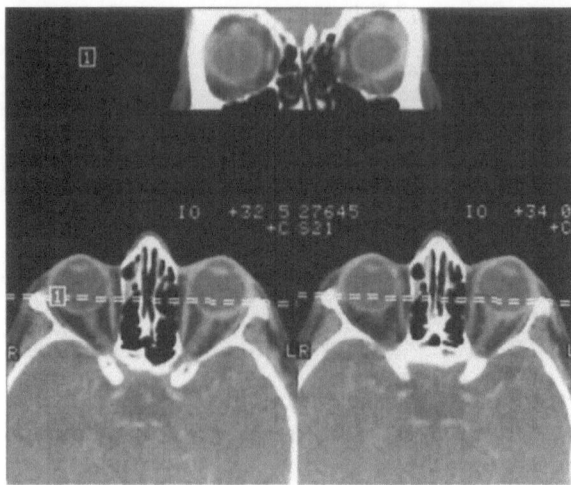

51.4

CT
Enlargement of the tendon of the left inferior oblique muscle, mainly at its insertion. Slight enlargement of the adjacent lacrimal gland.

Diagnosis
Scleritic-tenonitic form of inflammatory orbital
pseudotumor.

Clinical Course
Systemic steroid therapy (beginning with 100 mg
prednisolone, gradually reducing the dose) resulted in remission of signs and symptoms within
6 days.

Courtesy of Professor Hans Borgmann, Department of
Ophthalmology, Johanniter Hospital, Bonn, Germany.

K. G., 54-year-old man

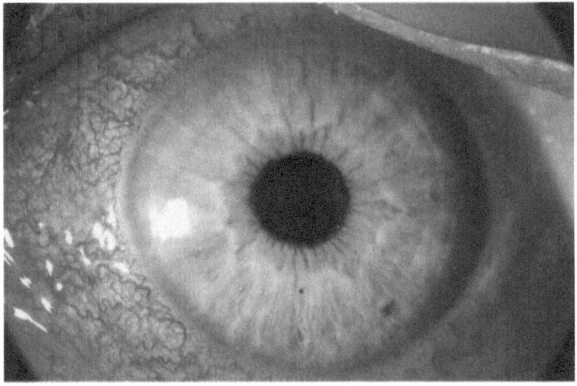

52.1

History and Clinical Findings
Severe pain in the area of the left eye, episcleral and scleral injection, periorbital swelling, and hyperemia for 3 days.

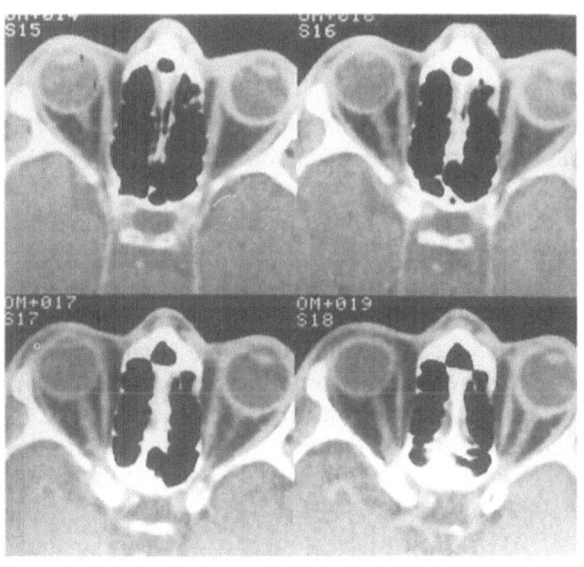

52.2

CT
Enlargement and contrast enhancement of the wall of the left globe.

Diagnosis
Scleritic-tenonitic form of inflammatory orbital pseudotumor.

Clinical Course
Fast and complete remission after systemic steroid therapy (beginning with 100 mg prednisolone, gradually reducing the dose).

D. B., 27-year-old woman

History and Clinical Findings
Acute onset of periorbital hyperemia and swelling 2 days ago, as well as severe pain in the area of the right eye.

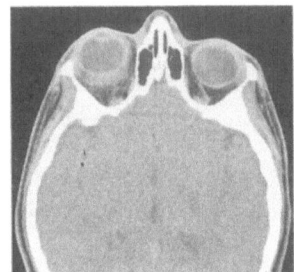

53.1

CT (53.1)
Enlargement of the wall of the right globe, infiltration of the adjacent retrobulbar space.

Diagnosis
Scleritic-tenonitic form of inflammatory orbital pseudotumor.

Clinical Course
Fast remission after systemic steroid therapy (beginning with 100 mg prednisolone, gradually reducing the dose).

CT (53.2)
No pathological CT findings after 3 weeks.

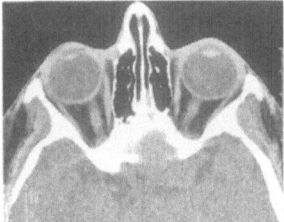

53.2

Dacryoadenitic Form of Inflammatory ▷ Orbital Pseudotumor

The dacryoadenitic form of inflammatory orbital pseudotumor usually occurs unilaterally and is accompanied by a massive, homogeneous swelling of the orbital and palpebral portion of the lacrimal gland. In some cases, the adjacent lateral rectus muscle may also be affected. The clinical signs are ptosis, hyperemia and swelling of the upper lid. Both, the ptosis and the swelling are temporally accentuated (Case 25).

Since its onset is so acute, the dacryoadenitic form of inflammatory orbital pseudotumor may be mistaken for acute bacterial dacryoadenitis. In the early stage, the diagnosis of bacterial dacryoadenitis is quite difficult to establish, especially if there are no typical signs of bacterial infection, such as purulent material or pathogenic bacteria in the conjunctival sac. Abscess formation within the lacrimal gland occurs usually in later stages. In bacterial dacryoadenitis the palpebral portion of the lacrimal gland is predominantly affected, while in inflammatory orbital pseudotumor the palpebral and orbital portions are usually equally affected.

In patients who have been or who are taking antibiotic medication, or in immunosuppressed patients, or in patients with infections with pathogens of low virulence, there are mitigated forms of bacterial dacryoadenitis. These forms are difficult to differentiate from the dacryoadenitic form of inflammatory orbital pseudotumor (Case 21). In these cases, CT visualization of abscesses in the palpebral portion of the lacrimal gland may facilitate the diagnosis.

A slowly progressive course of the dacryoadenitic form of inflammatory orbital pseudotumor cannot be differentiated by radiological means alone from other nonspecific inflammations, such as nonspecific dacryoadenitis, sarcoidosis, Wegener's granulomatosis, and Sjögren's syndrome, from leukemic infiltrations, or from the dacryoadenitic form of Graves' disease. Thorough medical examination, and possibly also a biopsy, are required to establish the diagnosis. In cases of diffuse inflammatory infiltration including the palpebral portion of the lacrimal gland, a biopsy of the palpebral portion using cocaine eye drops for anesthesia may be sufficient.

R. B., 24-year-old woman

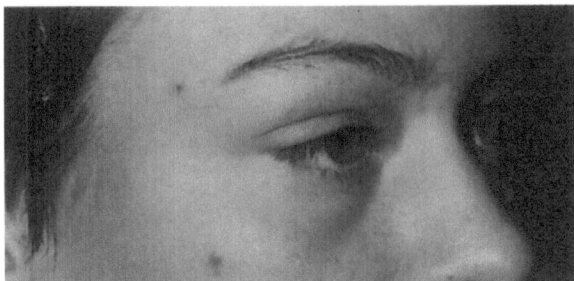

54.1

History and Clinical Findings
Painless swelling of the upper lid for 7 months.

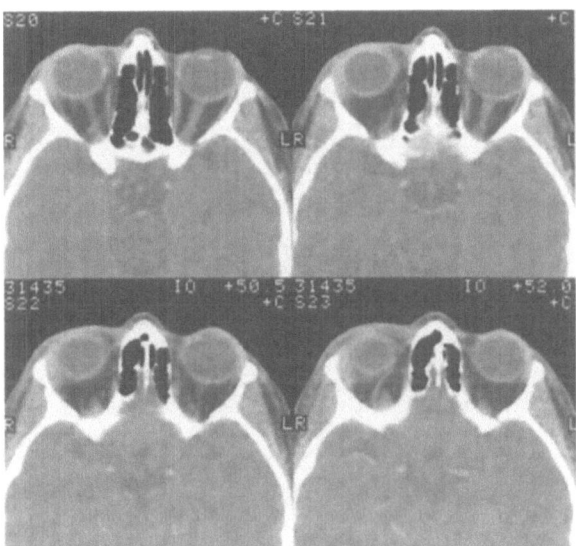

54.2

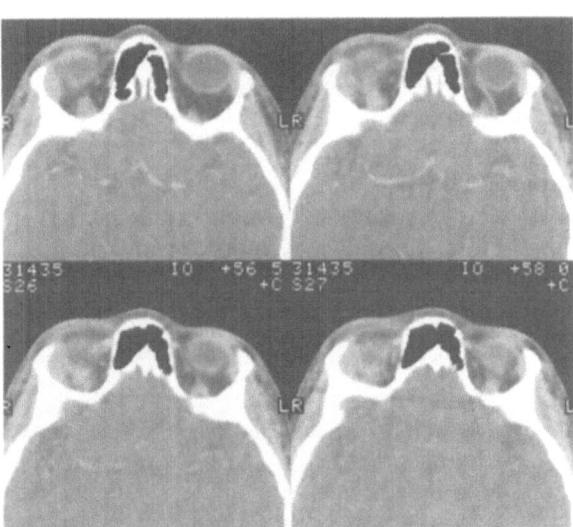

54.3

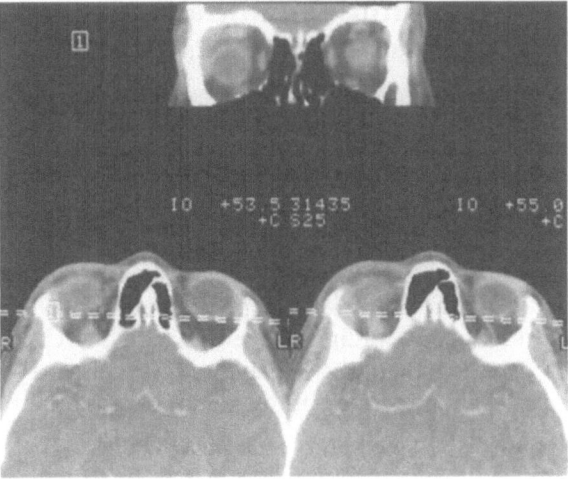

54.4

CT
Moderate enlargement of the right lacrimal gland and slight enlargement of the adjacent wall of the globe, as well as swelling of the upper lid.

Diagnosis
Dacryoadenitic form of inflammatory orbital pseudotumor. Concomitant swelling of the wall of the globe and the lid.

Moderate Diffusely Infiltrating Form of Inflammatory Orbital Pseudotumor

The moderate diffusely infiltrating form of inflammatory orbital pseudotumor is a combination of tenonitis, myositis of several extraocular muscles, and moderate infiltration of the orbital fat. Infiltration is observed at the margins of the Tenon's capsule and along the optic nerve sheath. Adjacent parts of the orbital fat appear hyperdense. This pattern of CT findings, together with the clinical picture, particularly its acute onset and severe pain, is characteristic of this form of inflammatory orbital pseudotumor.

P. R., 39-year-old woman

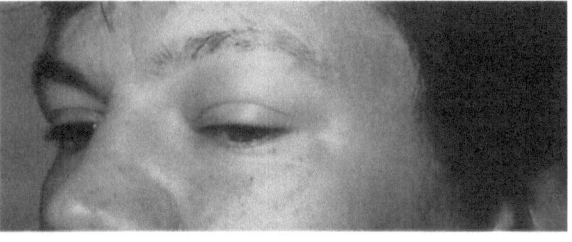

55.1

History and Clinical Findings
Increasing swelling of the left upper lid and a sensation of pressure behind the eye for the past 3 months.

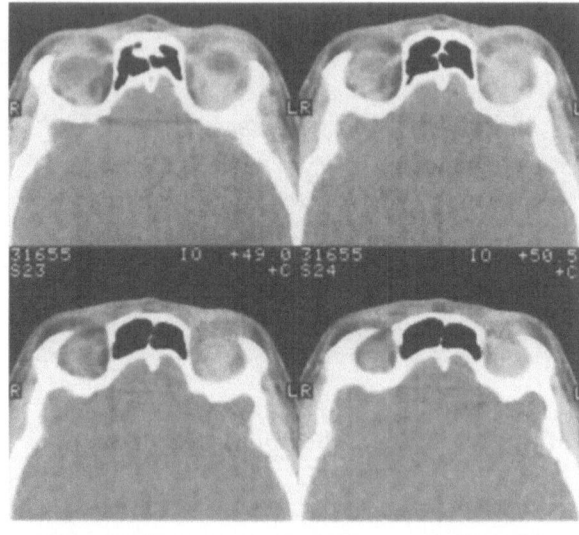

55.3

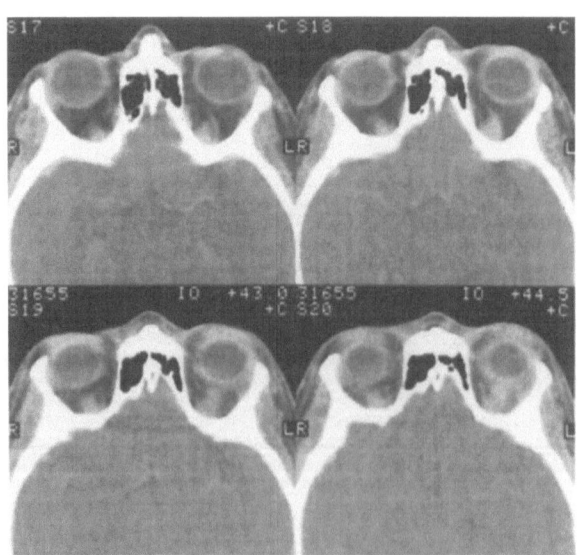

55.4

55.2

CT (55.2–55.4)
Diffuse infiltration of the left upper extraconal space, enlargement of the wall of the globe, considerable swelling of the upper lid, and slight proptosis.

Differential Diagnosis
Most probably, diffusely infiltrating form of inflammatory orbital pseudotumor and scleritis-tenonitis.

Systemic lymphatic disease must be excluded.

(Continued on p. 87)

Clinical Course

Clinical remission after steroid treatment (beginning with 100 mg prednisolone, gradually reducing the dose) within 8 days.

CT after 6 weeks: no pathological findings.

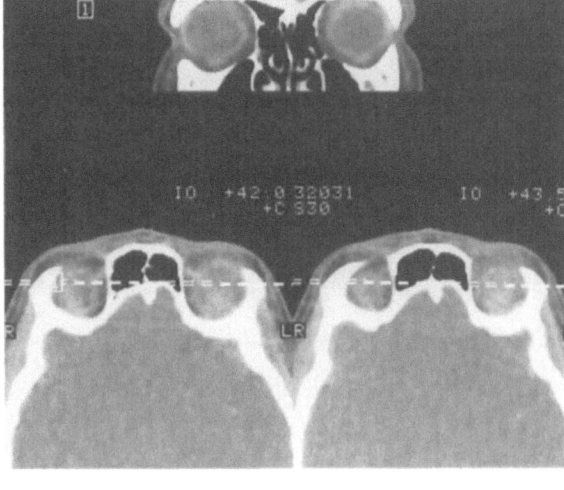

55.7

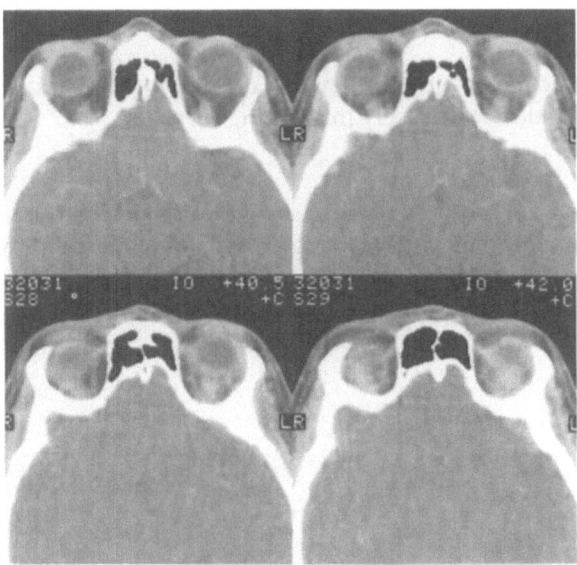

55.5

CT (55.5–55.7)

Only very few striated hyperdense areas within the upper extraconal fat.

Clinical Course

Recurrence 18 months later. Another 3 months later, the right orbit was affected (55.8).

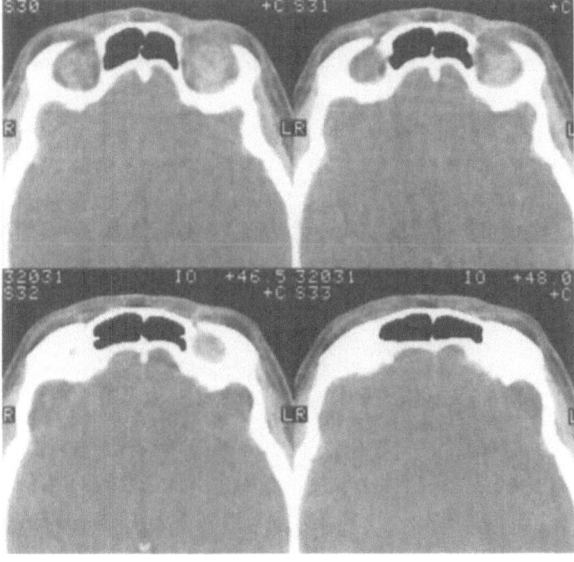

55.6

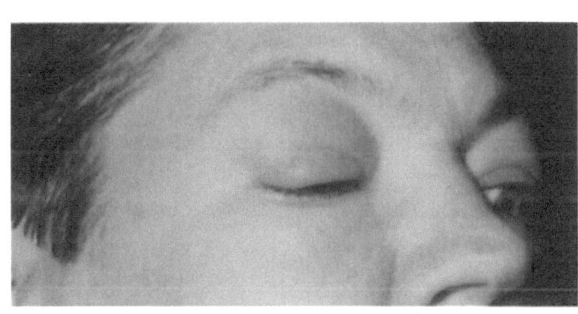

55.8

(Continued on p. 88)

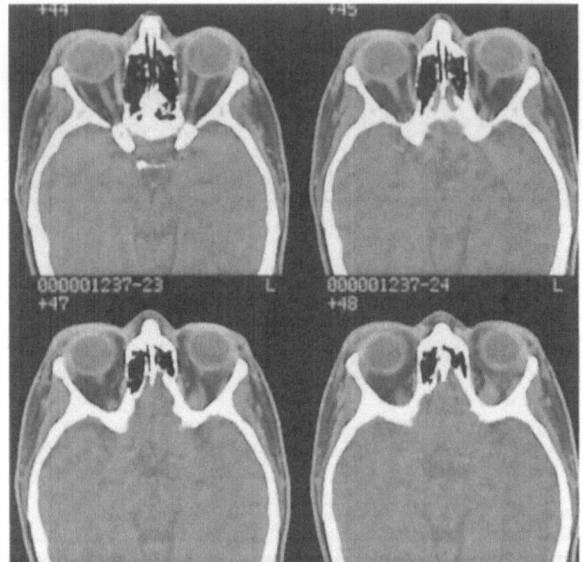

55.9

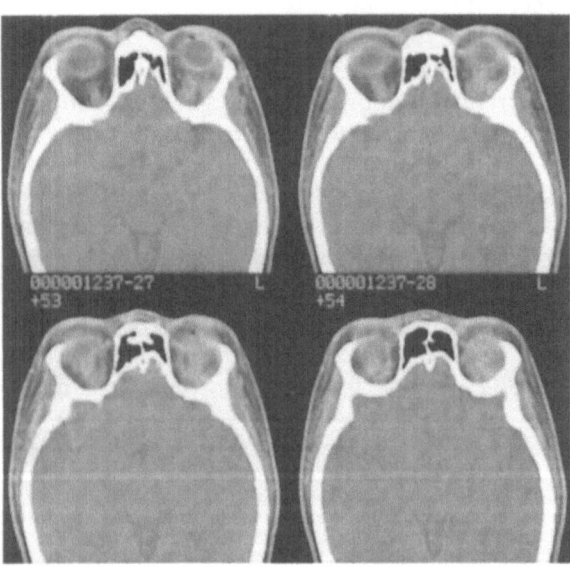

55.10

CT (55.9, 55.10):
Twenty-seven months later, increasing infiltration of the left upper extraconal space. Concomitant enlargement of the wall of the globe. Similar findings, but less pronounced, within the right upper extraconal space.

Diagnosis
Recurrent inflammatory orbital pseudotumor. Moderate diffusely infiltrating form.

Clinical Course
Again, good response to systemic steroid treatment (beginning with 100 mg prednisolone, gradually reducing the dose).

Systemic lymphatic disease was excluded.

N.R., 43-year-old woman

History and Clinical Findings
Two years ago, acute proptosis, ptosis and vertical diplopia. Initially, good response to steroid treatment, but several relapses after each discontinuation of treatment. Since the last relapse, long-term immunosuppressive therapy and continuation of low-dose steroids; no relapse after initiation of immunosuppressive therapy with azathioprine and continuation of low-dose steroids.

Presently intermittent exotropia with diplopia and 3 mm proptosis.

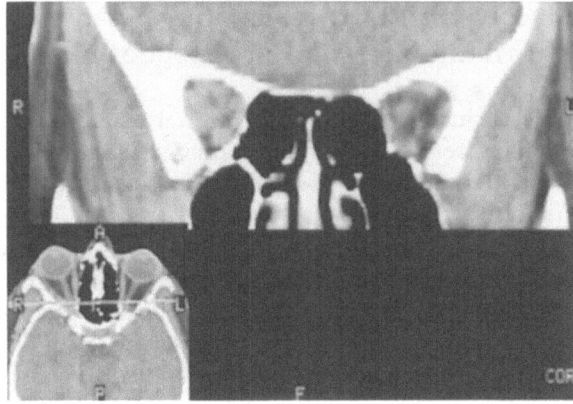

56.3

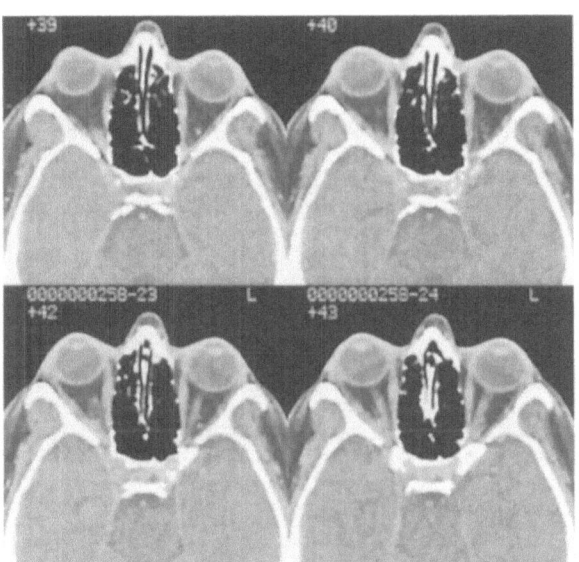

56.1

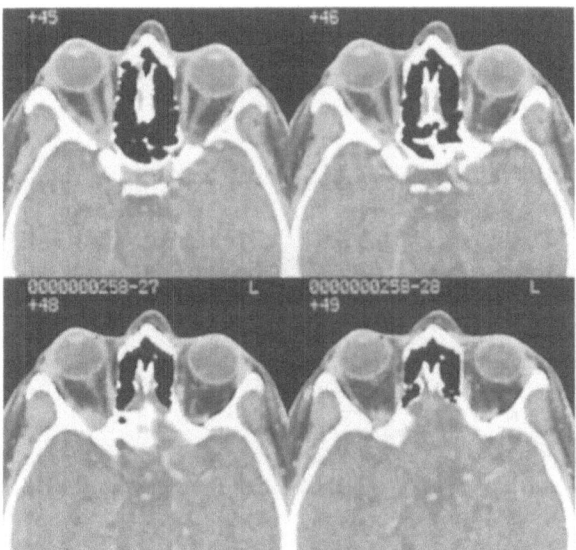

56.2

CT
Band-shaped, hyperdense area in the lateral part of the orbital apex, masking the lateral rectus muscle. No hyperostosis of the adjacent bone. Slight proptosis, slight enlargement of the ipsilateral cavernous sinus, extending into the superior orbital fissure. The right carotid artery cannot be delineated.

Diagnosis
Recurrence of the orbital pseudotumor. Infiltrating form of inflammatory orbital pseudotumor, extending into the cavernous sinus (Tolosa-Hunt syndrome).

Comment
Occlusion of the right internal carotid artery was confirmed by MRI-angiography and echography. Due to collateral circulation via the left basilar artery and the anterior cerebral arteries, blood supply was adequate.

Analysis of the CT scans alone does not allow confident differentiation from a meningioma. The fact that there is no hyperostosis, however, is not in favor of the diagnosis of a meningioma.

Massive Diffusely Infiltrating Form of Inflammatory Orbital Pseudotumor

This form of inflammatory orbital pseudotumor is characterized by inflammatory infiltration that is so dense that it completely masks all orbital structures.

This form cannot be distinguished from a dense, leukemic infiltration. Establishment of the diagnosis is mainly based on the clinical picture, characterized by acute onset and severe pain. This form of inflammatory orbital pseudotumor can be differentiated from orbital cellulitis due to sinusitis by visualization of nonaffected, air-filled paranasal sinuses. If the disease is taking a subacute course, a surgical biopsy is usually warranted.

S. J., 13-year-old girl

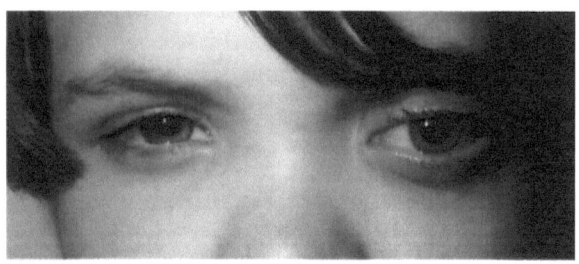

57.1

History and Clinical Findings
Increasing proptosis for the past 4 years. Slight reduction in visual acuity.

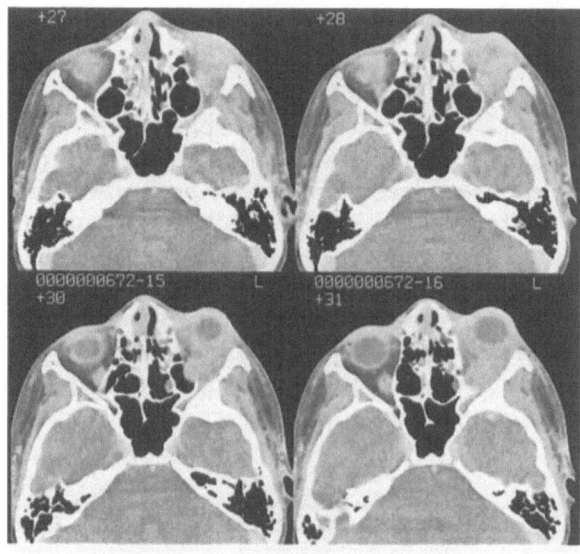

57.2

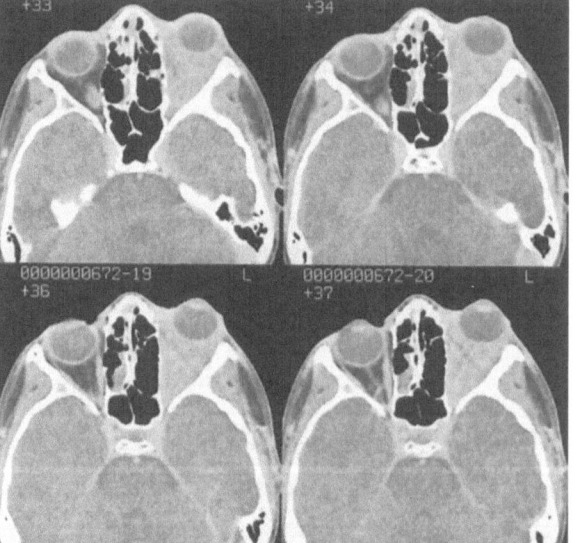

57.3

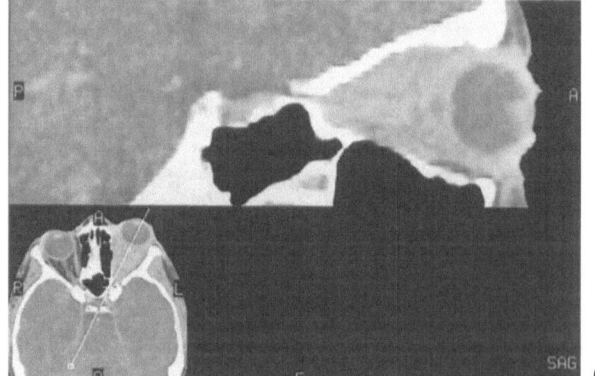

57.4

(Continued on p. 91)

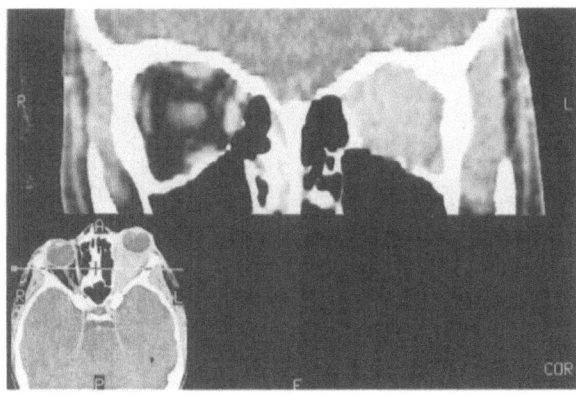

57.5

CT
Hyperostosis of the orbital walls. The orbit is filled with a homogenous soft-tissue mass, in which the optic nerve appears as a hypodense band. This mass surrounds and protrudes the globe, masking all other orbital structures. The orbital septum bulges out. Through a bone defect which has developed due to constant pressure, the tumor expands into the left maxillary sinus and into the inferior orbital fissure. Distention of the frontozygomatic suture. The cavernous sinus does not appear to be involved.

Diagnosis
Histopathologically confirmed inflammatory orbital pseudotumor (biopsy 2 years ago), massive diffusely infiltrating form.

Comment
Hyperostosis of the orbital walls and the smooth margins of the bone defects due to constant pressure offer evidence of a longstanding lesion, as well as evidence against an acute inflammatory or destructive lesion, or a lymphoma.

After failure of steroid treatment, anti-inflammatory radiation therapy is scheduled. In view of the patient's age, immunosuppressive therapy has been rejected.

Soft-Tissue Mass – Another Form of Inflammatory Orbital Pseudotumor

Another form of inflammatory orbital pseudo-tumor consists of a more or less well-delineated mass of soft tissue. The onset is usually less acute and not as painful as the diffusely infiltrating forms. Because it is not possible to differentiate the inflammatory mass from other soft-tissue tumors or metastases, a surgical biopsy is usually necessary. These tumors are frequently seen in patients with panarteritis nodosa. In patients with Wegener's granulomatosis, the origin of the soft-tissue masses is usually within paranasal sinuses or surrounding bone, from where it extends into the orbit. Since inflammatory granulomas are also observed in patients with other inflammatory diseases, such as tuberculosis, sarcoidosis, midline granuloma, etc. all patients with orbital soft-tissue masses need a complete medical examination and a surgical biopsy.

K. H., 73-year-old man

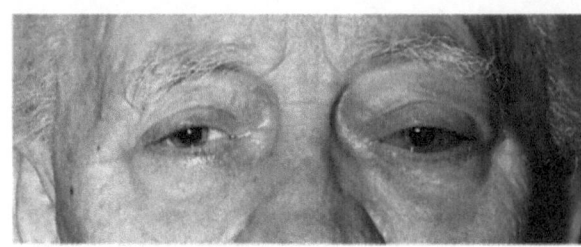

58.1

History and Clinical Findings
Rapidly increasing proptosis, periorbital swelling, ptosis, and chemosis.

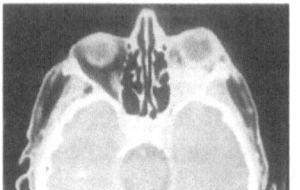

58.2

CT
Large soft-tissue mass within the intraconal space masking the adjacent orbital structures. Protrusion of the globe.

Differential Diagnosis
Inflammatory orbital pseudotumor or neoplasm.

Clinical Course
Rapid remission of signs and symptoms after systemic steroid treatment (beginning with 100 mg prednisolone, gradually reducing the dose).

Careful medical examination yielded no indication of malignancy or systemic inflammatory disease.

Inflammatory Orbital Pseudotumor Presenting as Aseptic Thrombophlebitis and Tolosa-Hunt Syndrome

Aseptic thrombophlebitis, a particular form of inflammatory orbital pseudotumor, occurring in the posterior orbital veins and sometimes extending into the cavernous sinus, usually leads to painful ophthalmoplegia. On CT scans, enlargement of the cavernous sinus and often also of the adjacent veins, which exhibit a hypodense lumen, the CT sign of thrombosis, can be visualized. Piercing pain in the ipsilateral side of the head, ophthalmoplegia, and usually a rapid response to steroid treatment are characteristic clinical features (Borgmann 1983).

Similar signs and symptoms, however, are brought about by aneurysms of the internal carotid and ophthalmic arteries, as well as by metastases within the cavernous sinus, and sometimes by parasellar tumors, such as adenomas of the pituitary gland and chordomas. Thorough neuroradiological examinations to exclude a malignant neoplasm must always be performed. The diagnosis of Tolosa-Hunt syndrome can only be established by exclusion: required are a clinical course of several years, and repeated, rapid responses to steroid treatment, as well as negative radiographic findings.

Metastases may also respond to steroid treatment, so that any improvement of symptoms may be misinterpreted as confirmation of the diagnosis of Tolosa-Hunt syndrome. If, after reduction or discontinuation of treatment, symptoms recur, this may be interpreted as the typical relapsing nature of the Tolosa-Hunt syndrome. In the beginning of the relapsing course of this syndrome, the diagnosis cannot be established with certainty. Follow-up at short intervals is therefore crucial, especially since neoplastic infiltrations or primary tumors of the cavernous sinus can often only be visualized after several months.

Another differential diagnosis to be considered is fungal infection of the sphenoid sinus. Since fungi may grow "en plaque" along the mucosa, they may easily escape detection. On CT and MRI scans one must specifically look for a possible thickening of the mucous membranes in the sphenoid sinuses and ethmoidal air cells or of the adjacent dura, as well as for incipient delicate bone destruction,

which is characteristic of longstanding fungal infections. In fungal infections steroid therapy may initially reduce pain but will eventually exacerbate the underlying disease.

R.L., 56-year-old woman

History and Clinical Findings
Intermittent, acute onset of severe pain in the supply area of the first branch of the left trigeminal nerve for the past 2 years.

Pain could be relieved only by strong analgesics. Painful attacks occurred at approximately weekly intervals.

Subsequent ipsilateral abducent nerve palsy, followed by complete oculomotor nerve palsy; both improved with steroid treatment, while visual function was reduced to 20/100 with a corresponding central scotoma.

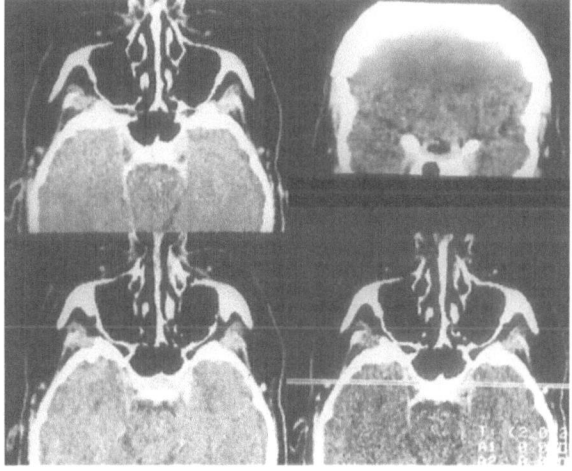

59.1–2

CT
Slight enlargement of the left cavernous sinus, which, compared with the right, appears hyperdense.

Differential Diagnosis
Suspicion of Tolosa-Hunt syndrome.
   A neoplastic infiltration must be excluded.

Comment
The diagnosis of Tolosa-Hunt syndrome is further substantiated by the 3-year clinical course with intermittent painful ophthalmoplegia, complete remission after each course of steroid treatment, and by the fact that no primary malignant neoplasm was found.

Courtesy of Professor Hans Borgmann, Department of Ophthalmology, Johanniter Hospital, Bonn, Germany.

5 Inflammatory Diseases of the Lacrimal Gland

Inflammations of the lacrimal gland lead to a swelling of the temporal part of the upper lid due to the gland's position in the upper and outer quadrant of the orbit with the palpebral portion within the lateral upper lid's conjunctiva. The lid swelling resembles a paragraph sign (page 45, Plate 12). It can be of acute onset due to an inflammatory orbital pseudotumor, bacterial dacryoadenitis, or a subperiosteal abscess and is often quite painful. Bacterial dacryoadenitis may result in necrosis and abscess formation, which either drain spontaneously or have to be treated surgically.

Slowly progressive dacryoadenitis often manifests in nothing more than moderate ptosis and diffuse swelling of the outer and upper lid and clinically cannot be distinguished from other cellular infiltrations, for instance infiltrations in lymphoma, metastases or histiocytosis X (Case 21).

Since the lacrimal glands are situated close to the aponeurosis of the levator palpebrae and the superior lateral rectus muscles, as well as to the conjunctiva and the sclera, primary inflammation of these tissues often involves the lacrimal glands. Since the lacrimal glands are well vascularized, they are highly susceptible to involvement in systemic viral diseases, such as epidemic parotitis and infectious mononucleosis, or adenovirus infections, e.g., epidemic keratoconjunctivitis. The high degree of vascularization also facilitates the deposition of neoplastic or leukemic cells.

The lacrimal gland is also quite often the first site to manifest autoimmune disease, for example Sjögren syndrome.

Other generalized inflammations, mainly those associated with collagen vascular disease, are characterized by infiltrations of the lacrimal glands by immune cells and infiltrations of other exocrine glands (parotid and submandibular glands, pancreas). The pathogenesis of this group of inflammations is not yet fully elucidated. Preceding viral infections, such as infections by the Epstein-Barr virus, may have a trigger function.

In Graves' disease the lacrimal gland is frequently affected. In some cases (dacryoadenitic form) it may be the only orbital structure affected. Glandular enlargement, however, can also be observed accompanying the swelling of extraocular muscles.

As the anterior portion of the lacrimal gland lies directly upon the aponeurosis of the levator palpebrae, this muscle is often unilaterally enlarged in patients with unilateral dacryoadenitis. Migration of inflammatory cells into the muscle first leads to ptosis and lid lag. The ensuing fibrosis may then cause persistent lid retraction. The other extraocular muscles appear normal. Scar formation within the levator palpebrae can be observed during plastic surgery of lid retraction. With increasing fibrosis, the enlarged muscle shrinks and the muscle belly may appear normal or even reduced in size.

Differential Diagnosis

Acute or chronic infiltration by inflammatory or neoplastic cells results in unilateral or bilateral diffuse enlargement of the entire gland while its almond shape is retained.

Differentiation between acute bacterial and nonspecific dacryoadenitis, as in viral disease or inflammatory orbital pseudotumor, requires examination for additional clinical signs such as purulent material in the conjunctival sac, fever, and leukocytosis. CT visualization of a possible abscess, a low-density area surrounded by a hyperdense margin in contrast-enhanced scans, or evidence of a subperiosteal abscess originating from an opacified sinus gives important clues for further differentiation.

If the infiltration of the lacrimal gland is inflammatory or leukemic in origin, enlargement is usually homogeneous. The lacrimal gland nestles closely to the globe. Primary epithelial neoplasms, i.e., mixed tumors, carcinomas, and carcinomas within mixed tumors, as well as metastases of carcinomas, almost invariably cause localized glandular enlargement.

Chronic systemic inflammatory disease and secondary scar formation may, by fibrosis, eventually also lead to deformation of the lacrimal gland, sometimes even with an indentation of the neighboring parts of the globe.

Because of the slow rate of growth, the mixed tumors of the lacrimal gland often cause excavation and thinning of neighboring bone, while primary and secondary carcinomas of the lacrimal gland infiltrate and erode the adjacent bone.

An important criterion for differentiating inflammatory fibrosing lesions from primary neoplasms is the unilateral occurrence of primary epithelial neoplasms of the lacrimal gland. Differentiating inflammatory fibrosing processes from metastases in the lacrimal gland is difficult, since they both may occur unilaterally as well as bilaterally. In many cases, the origin of lacrimal gland enlargement can only be identified by surgical biopsy. This particularly applies to distinguishing inflammatory from neoplastic, mostly leukemic, infiltrations, such as in lymphomas, histiocytosis X, etc. A lesion which is suggestive of a benign mixed tumor of the lacrimal gland, however, must not be biopsied.

"Patients who underwent a biopsy prior to excision of their benign mixed tumor had a five year recurrence rate of 32%, compared to the overall recurrence rate of 13%, while patients whose tumor was removed with the capsule intact had a five year recurrence rate of only 3%." (Font and Gamel 1978)

The most important criteria of benign mixed tumors are: a slowly progressive course, usually over many years, which may be documented by photographs; focal enlargement of the lacrimal gland impressing upon the globe; unilaterality of the lesion; and erosion of the adjacent bone. If any one of the above mentioned criteria is met, no biopsy must be performed but a primary en-bloc resection including the adjacent bone is imperative.

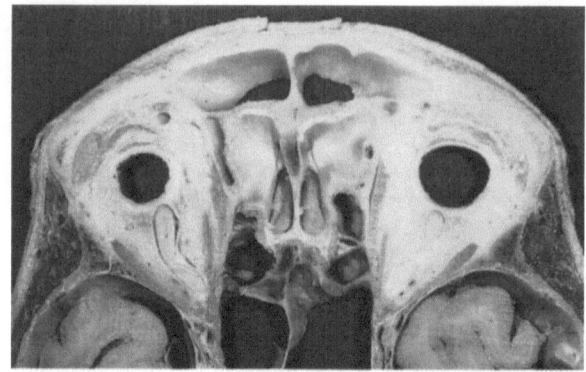

60.1

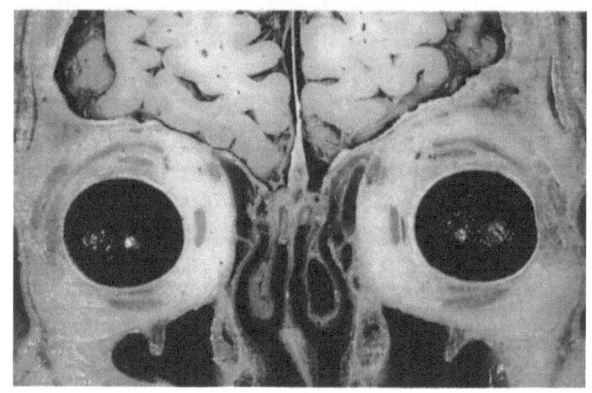

60.2

Axial and coronal anatomical section through the lacrimal gland.

Note location of the lacrimal gland in the superior and anterior temporal part of the orbit directly on the aponeurosis of the levator palpebrae muscle. (Courtesy of Professor Jack DeGroot, former Chief of Neuroanatomy, Department of Anatomy, University of California Medical School, San Francisco, California, USA)

K.F.-G., 11-year-old boy

History and Clinical Finding
Infectious mononucleosis 5 months ago, varicella 3 months ago. For 2 days, increasing swelling of the right upper lid and periorbital hyperemia. Moderate conjunctival injection. No pathogenic bacteria isolated in the conjunctival smear. No pathological findings on ENT examination.

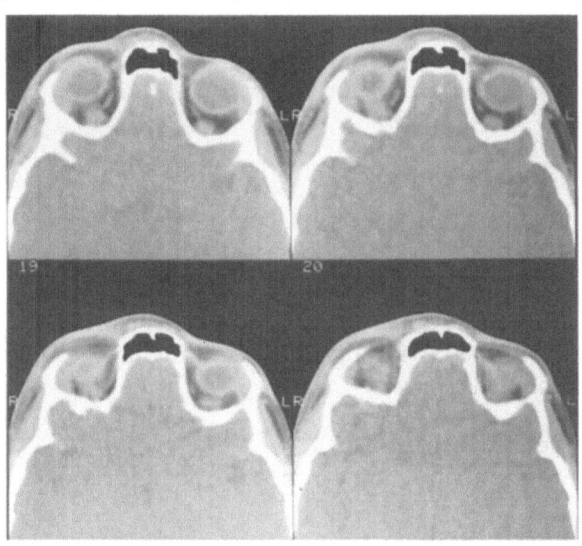

61.1

CT
Minor, homogeneous enlargement of the lacrimal gland, slight swelling of the right upper lid.

Diagnosis
Acute dacryoadenitis, most likely of viral origin.

Clinical Course
With regard to systemic inflammatory disease or bacterial infection, no pathological findings in laboratory immunological examinations.

Spontaneous, complete remission of all clinical findings within a period of 5 days.

F. K., 66-year-old man

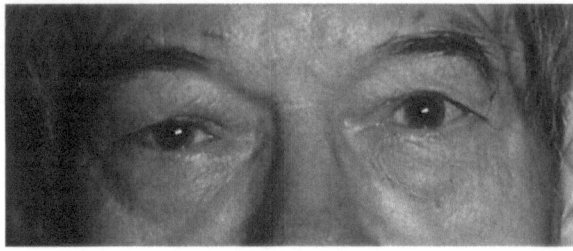

62.1

History and Clinical Findings
Intermittent ptosis and swelling of the right upper lid for the past 4 months. Now moderate swelling and ptosis. Slight conjunctival injection and enlargement of the palpebral portion of the lacrimal gland.

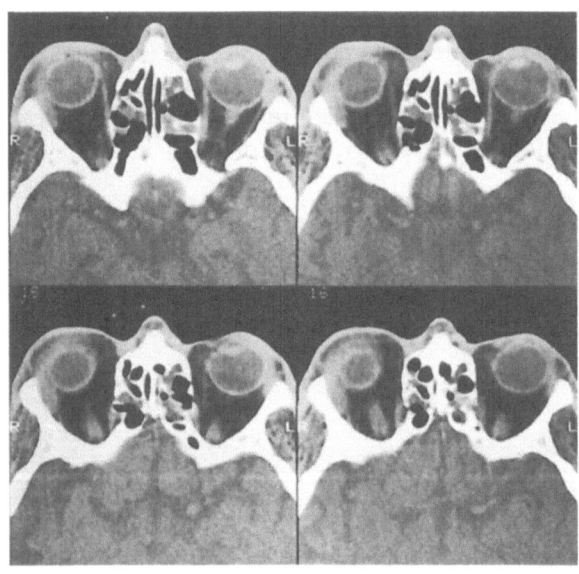

62.2

CT
Edema of the upper lid and homogeneous enlargement of the lacrimal gland, extending far into the retrobulbar space.

Differential Diagnosis
Chronic inflammatory or neoplastic infiltration.

Clinical Course
Surgical biopsy: dense infiltration by plasma cells and lymphocytes, hyperplastic chronic inflammatory reaction, consistent with inflammatory orbital pseudotumor.

Increased synthesis of monoclonal immunoglobulins within regional plasma cells requires consideration of an early stage of lymphoma. Medical and laboratory examinations yielded no indication of systemic disease.

K. M., 30-year-old man

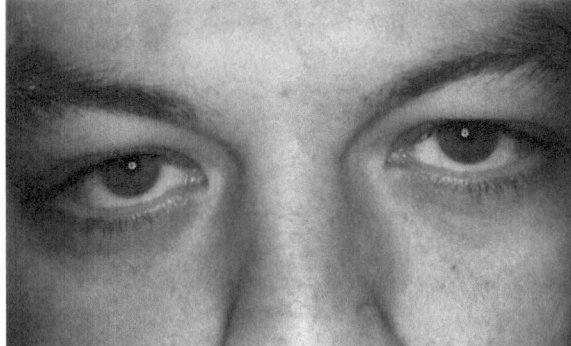

63.1

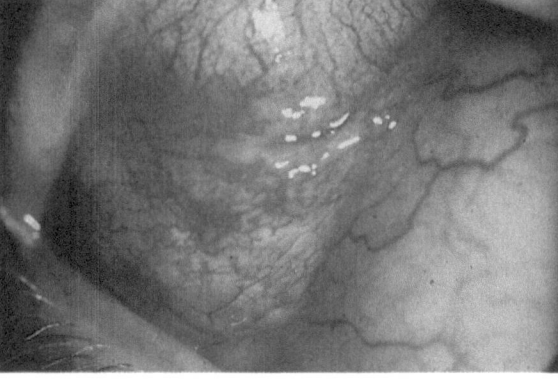

63.2

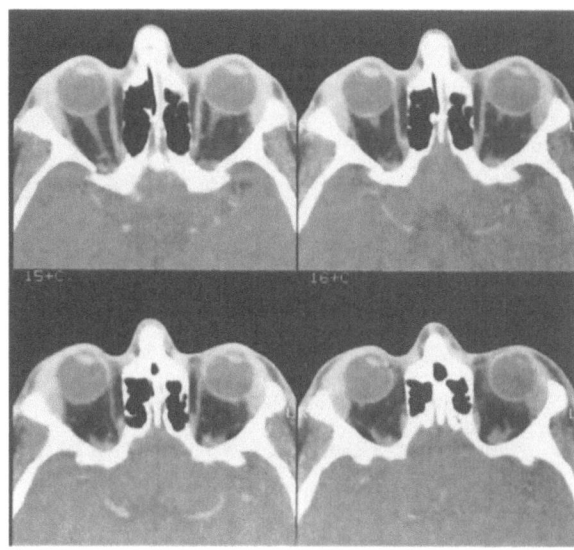

63.4

History and Clinical Findings

For the past 4 weeks, swelling of both upper lids and painful swelling of the right ankle joint. Because of transient conjunctivitis and dysuria, Reiter's syndrome was suspected, but HLA B27 typing was negative. Remission of signs and symptoms with steroid therapy. After discontinuation of steroid treatment, recurrence of arthritis and lid swelling.

CT

Considerable enlargement of both lacrimal glands.

Differential Diagnosis

Chronic dacryoadenitis, probably due to systemic inflammatory disease.

Clinical Course

Surgical biopsy: chronic, sclerosing and atrophying dacryoadenitis, no signs of sarcoidosis.

Medical examination yielded no indication of systemic inflammatory disease.

Diagnosis

HLA B27-negative arthritis and bilateral chronic dacryoadenitis.

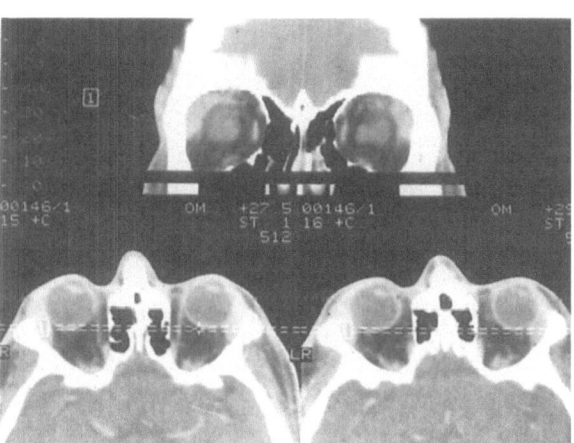

63.3

K. L., 19-year-old woman

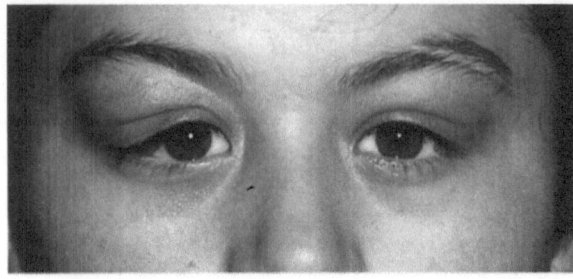

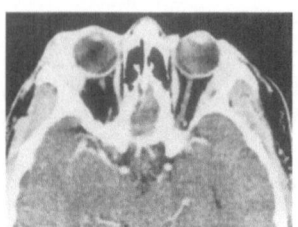

64.3

64.1

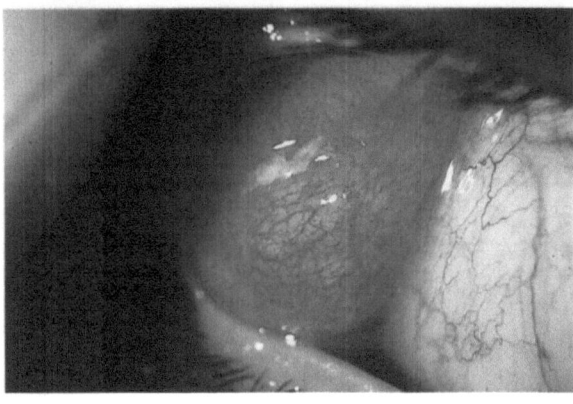

64.2

CT
Considerable homogeneous enlargement of both lacrimal glands extending both anteriorly and posteriorly into the extraconal space.

Diagnosis
Recurrent bilateral dacryoadenitis.

Clinical Course
In view of the patient's age, and despite the patient's wish, no anti-inflammatory or immunosuppressive treatment was initiated. Complete remission during pregnancy 18 months later (64.4). No relapse since then (follow-up for 5 years).

History and Clinical Findings
Recurrent, acute bouts of swelling of both lacrimal glands. Massive swelling and hyperemia of the temporal parts of both upper lids. When the patient gazes downward and the upper lid is lifted, the inflamed and swollen palpebral portion of the lacrimal gland bulges out (64.2).

Thorough medical and laboratory immunological examinations yielded no signs of systemic inflammatory disease, particularly no indication of Sjögren's syndrome.

Histopathology
Dense infiltration by lymphocytes and plasma cells.

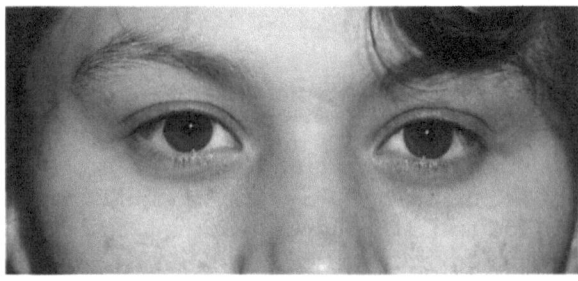
64.4

S. G., 41-year-old man

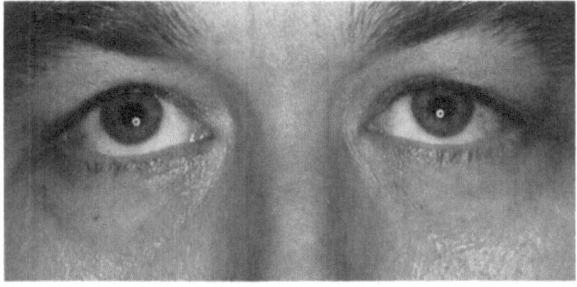

65.1

History and Clinical Findings
For the past 3 months, slight bilateral ptosis and swelling of the temporal upper lids, no hyperemia. Sensation of pressure in the anterior and temporal parts of the orbit.

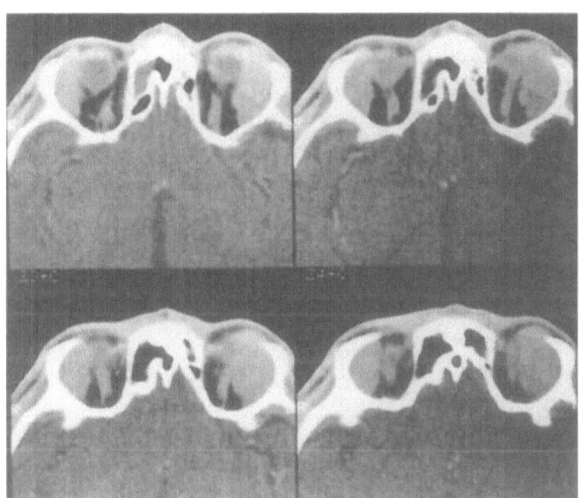

65.2

CT
Massive homogeneous enlargement of both lacrimal glands, extending far into the lateral and superior extraconal space. The globes are medially and inferiorly displaced.

Diagnosis
Bilateral chronic dacryoadenitis.

Histopathology
Inflammatory infiltration of the lacrimal gland, predominantly by lymphocytes and plasma cells.

Clinical Course
Later, development of bilateral parotitis and a pancreatic tumor.

Histopathology (pancreas): chronic nonspecific inflammation.

Partial removal of the lacrimal gland (elsewhere): identical histopathology.

S. B., 71-year-old man

History and Clinical Findings
Bilateral swelling of the upper lid for 18 months.

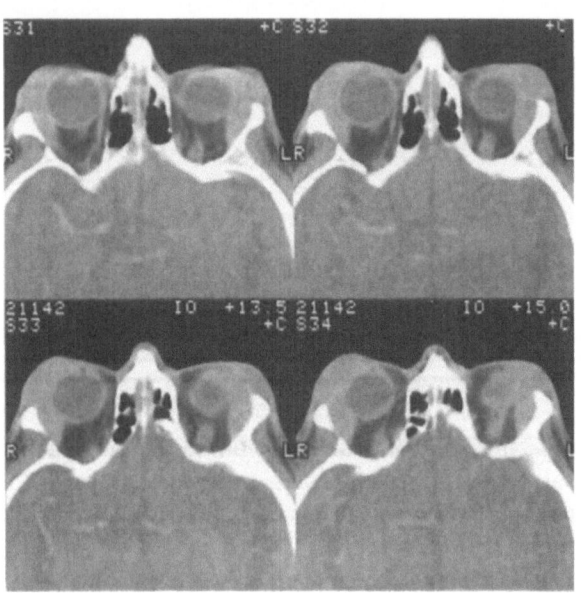

66.1

CT
Massive, symmetrical enlargement of both lacrimal glands, extending far into the lateral and superior extraconal space. Displacement of both lateral rectus muscles. No displacement and no impression of the globe.

Diagnosis
Suspected lymphatic disease.

Clinical Course
Low-grade non-Hodgkin's lymphoma (suspected MALT lymphoma). Malignant gastric lymphoma of the stomach had been treated with radiotherapy 6 years previously, followed by complete remission.

Comment
Considering the very slight clinical inflammatory signs as well as the symmetry of all CT findings, the acute dacryoadenitic form of inflammatory orbital pseudotumor is an unlikely diagnosis.

Computed tomography does not permit differentiation from leukemic infiltrations or other systemic inflammatory disease.

E. C., 22-year-old man

History and Clinical Findings
Extraocular muscle surgery 4 days ago. Progressive swelling of the right upper lid and slight proptosis. Progression of lid edema and chemosis despite systemic antibiotic treatment.

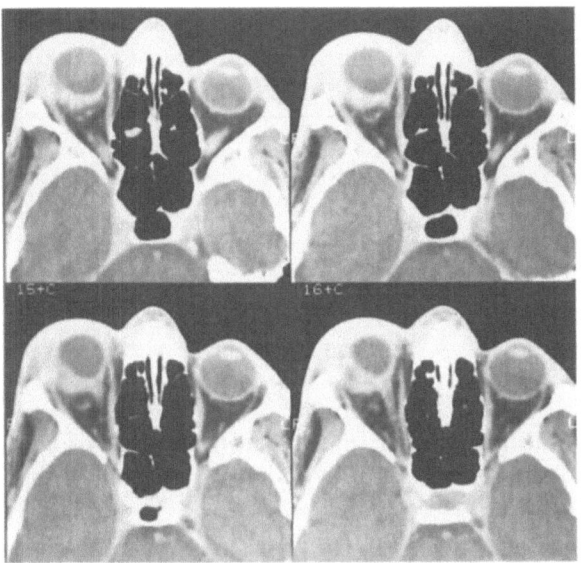

67.1

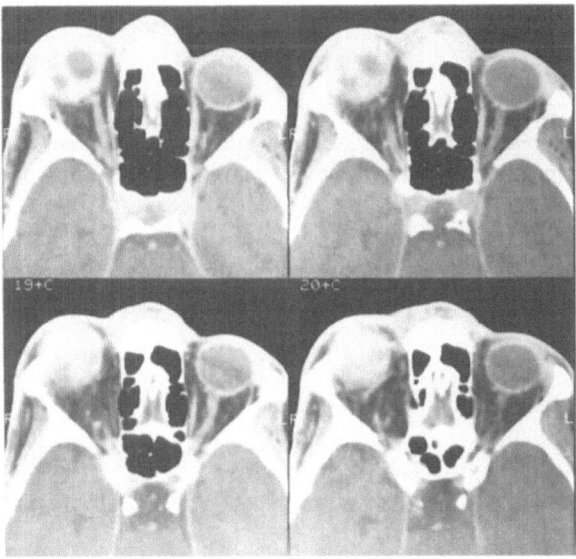

7.2

CT
Considerable enlargement of the wall of the right globe and of the eye lids. Moderate enlargement of the right lacrimal gland with several hypodense areas of different size. Enlarged retrobulbar veins appear as striate areas of increased density within the orbital fat.

Diagnosis
Postoperative abscesses within the right lacrimal gland.

Clinical Course
Abscess drainage, followed by rapid remission of signs and symptoms.

M. D., 28-year-old man

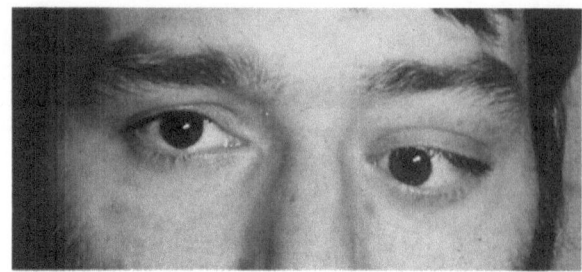

68.1

Typical aspect of a slowly growing tumor of the lacrimal gland. The globe is displaced inferiorly, medially, and anteriorly. Previous photos show that proptosis had developed over a period of 5 years. The slow development points to a mixed tumor of the lacrimal gland.

Histopathology
Mixed tumor of the lacrimal gland (pleomorphic adenoma).

S. R., 31-year-old woman

History and Clinical Findings
Swelling of the right upper lid for 6 weeks. No pain. Diplopia in right gaze.

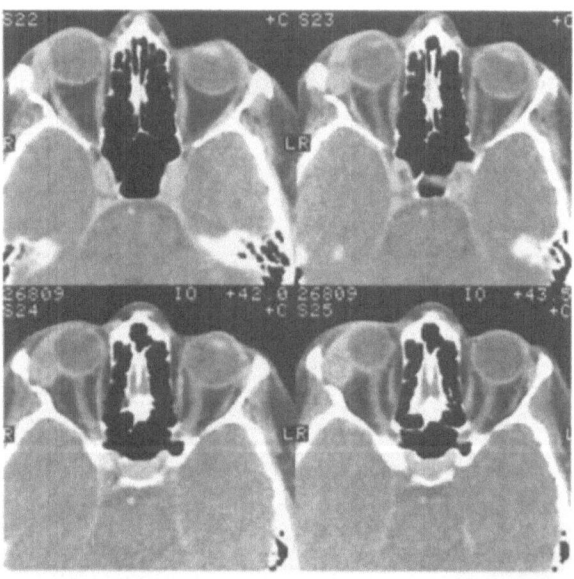

69.1

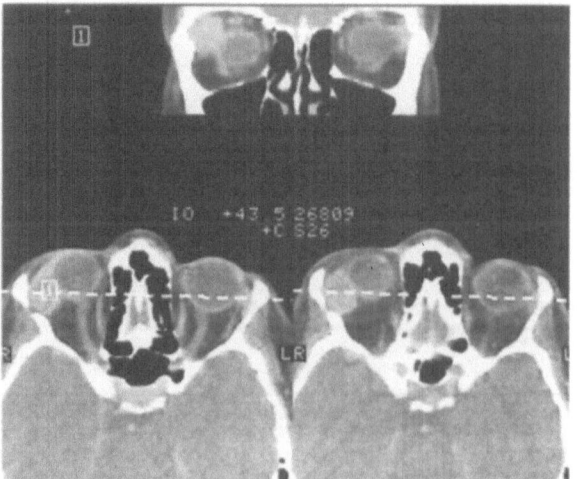

69.2

CT
Well-defined enlargement of the right lacrimal gland. Erosion of the adjacent lateral orbital wall. Proptosis. Small hypodense areas within the tumor.

Diagnosis
Mixed tumor of the lacrimal gland. Malignancy cannot be excluded.

Surgery
Mixed tumor of the lacrimal gland (pleomorphic adenoma).

Comment
Excavation of the bone indicates slowly progressive growth of the tumor.

S. I., 41-year-old woman

History and Clinical Findings
The patient reports removal of a tumor in the area of the right lacrimal gland 6 years ago. During the past year, swelling of the right upper lid. Surgical biopsy of a tumor of the lacrimal gland 2 months ago.

CT
Space-occupying lesion in the right lacrimal gland. The upper muscle complex cannot be clearly delineated.

Differential Diagnosis
Malignant tumor of the lacrimal gland suspected.

Clinical Course
Osteoplastic trepanation of the lateral and superior orbital wall and exenteration of the orbit.

Histopathology
Adenoid-cystic carcinoma of the lacrimal gland.

Comment
The initial operation should have been performed as an en-bloc resection. It remains unclear whether the primary tumor was a benign mixed tissue tumor which underwent malignant transformation, or whether the tumor primarily contained carcinomatous parts.

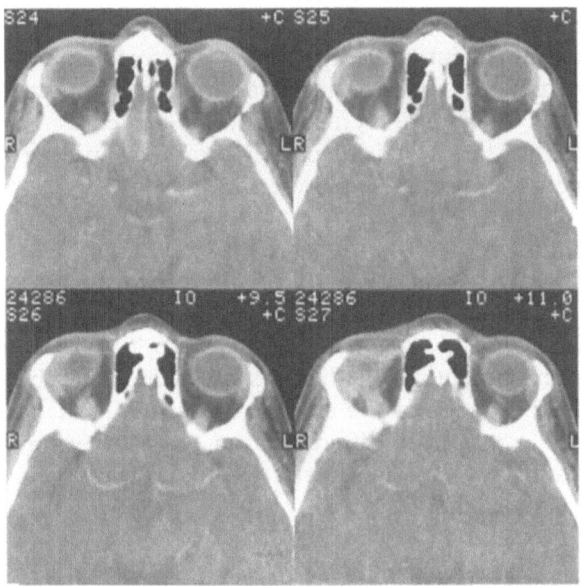

70.1

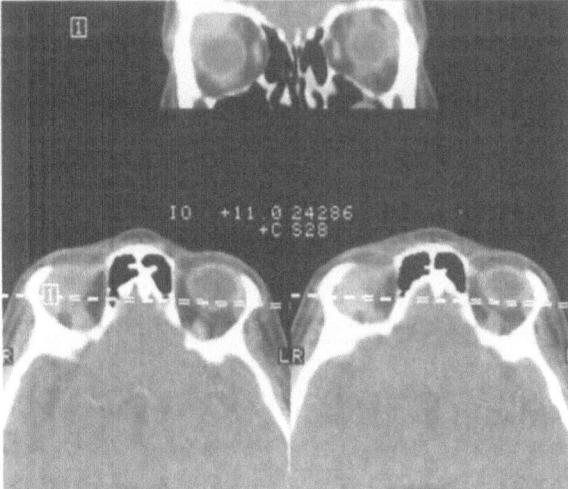

70.2

S. G., 66-year-old woman

History and Clinical Findings
Mastectomy and subsequent radiation therapy
6 years ago. Metastases into skin and lungs.
  Ptosis and diplopia for the past 4 weeks.

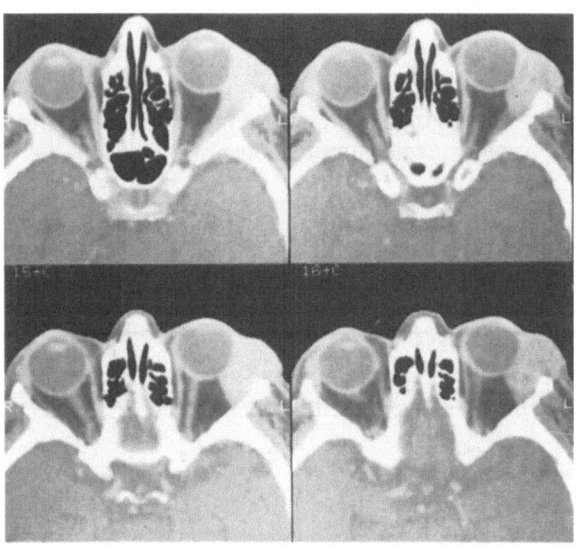

71.1

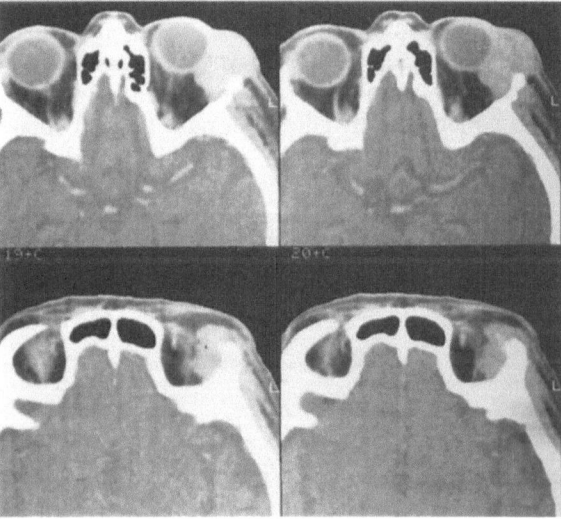

71.2

CT
In the area of the left lacrimal gland a vast, largely
homogeneous, polycyclic space-occupying lesion,
bulging far into both the anterior extraconal and
retrobulbar space. The adjacent bone appears
intact. The lateral rectus muscle can be delineated
clearly. The globe is displaced anteriorly and medially, the lateral wall is indented.

Diagnosis
Metastasis of the known carcinoma of the breast.

Comment
Establishment of the diagnosis was facilitated by
the knowledge of the clinical situation. CT alone
does not permit differentiation from other inflammatory and neoplastic lesions affecting the
lacrimal gland.

B. T., 14-year-old boy

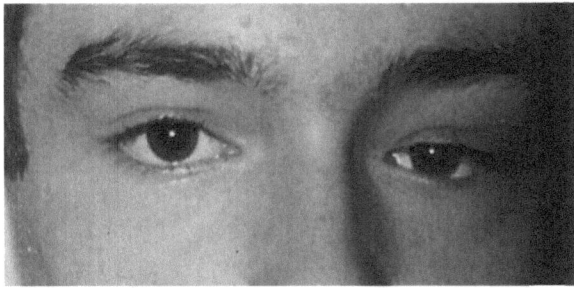

72.1

History and Clinical Findings
Minor head trauma 3 weeks ago. Since then progressive, temporally accentuated hyperemia, swelling of the upper lid, ptosis, and downward displacement of the left globe.

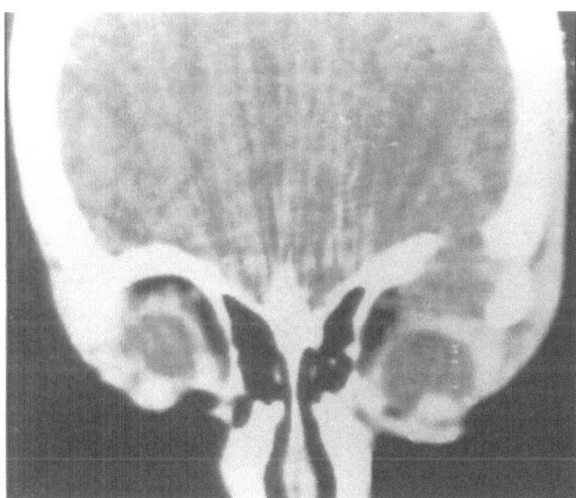

72.2

CT
A large part of the left orbital roof has been destroyed in its entire width by a soft-tissue mass extending into the orbit and displacing the globe.

Diagnosis
Suspicion of histiocytosis X ("eosinophilic granuloma").

Histopathology
Histiocytosis X.

Clinical Course
Rapid remission of clinical signs and symptoms after local radiation therapy.

Comment
While the clinical appearance does not allow conclusions as to the nature of the lesion (cf. p. 45, Plate 12), characteristic CT findings – a large defect through the entire bone with an adjacent soft-tissue mass is typical – and knowledge of the patient's age allow the diagnosis of histiocytosis X (esosinophilic granuloma) to be established with a high degree of safety.

6 Orbital Inflammations Secondary to Paranasal Sinus Disease and Their Differential Diagnoses

With the exception of the lateral wall, the orbit is surrounded by paranasal sinuses (Fig. 73a): medially by the ethmoidal air cells and the sphenoid sinus, inferiorly by the maxillary sinus, and superiorly by the frontal sinus. The anterior-superior parts of the sphenoidal sinus are situated medially to the optic canal. Depending on the degree of pneumatization, the paranasal sinus and the orbit share broad boundaries. This is why lesions of the paranasal sinuses so often affect the orbit. Inflammations and neoplasms may destroy the in part very thin bony barriers, such as the lamina papyracea, and spread underneath the periosteum into the orbital cavity, for instance in bacterial sinusitis (Case 75), Wegener's granulomatosis (Case 77), mucoceles, and mucopyoceles. The latter may develop spontaneously, after trauma or surgery, or due to neoplastic lesions obstructing a sinus' ostium. For diagnosing sinus lesions with orbital involvement, thin-section CT has proven to be the examination method of choice, as intraorbital soft-tissue lesions and bone destructions can be visualized equally well.

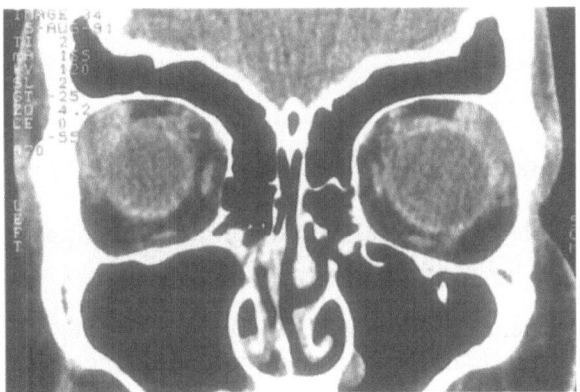

73a

Figure 73 a

Coronal CT section through the anterior orbit: excessive pneumatization of the paranasal sinuses augments the extension of common boundaries with the orbit.

Orbital Complications of Bacterial Sinusitis

Bacterial infections of the paranasal sinuses may lead to severe and at times life-threatening complications. In children accumulation of purulent discharge occurs mainly within the ethmoidal air cells; in adults complications also arise from frontal and, less often, from maxillary sinus infections. Infectious material can spread from the paranasal sinus via the ethmoidal veins and the superior ophthalmic vein to the cavernous sinus (Case 73c). Septic cavernous sinus thrombosis is still a life-threatening situation. Septic material may also be transmitted via the anterior ethmoidal veins to the anterior meningeal vein, where it may cause frontal cerebral abscesses.

The clinical picture of orbital involvement in bacterial sinusitis is generally characterized by periorbital hyperemia and swelling, narrowing of the palpebral fissure, and proptosis. Septic thrombophlebitis of orbital veins is usually the earliest stage of orbital involvement in infectious sinus disease, before a subperiosteal abscess forms or purulent material spreads into the orbital cavity.

The clinical aspect of the different orbital complications of infectious sinus disease is nonspecific. Septic thrombophlebitis cannot be distinguished from the other complications, such as subperiosteal abscess, incipient thrombosis of the cavernous sinus, penetration of septic material into the orbit, or unspecific, noninfectious inflammations such as inflammatory orbital pseudotumor. It should be kept in mind that many different pathological processes may present similar clinical aspects, especially in the examination of children: inflammatory reactions can be the first sign of a rapidly growing neoplasm, such as rhabdomyosarcoma, neuroblastoma, or histiocytosis X (cf. p. 45, Plate 12).

When patients present with periorbital hyperemia and edema, restricted eye movement, ptosis and proptosis, one should refrain from a "clinical

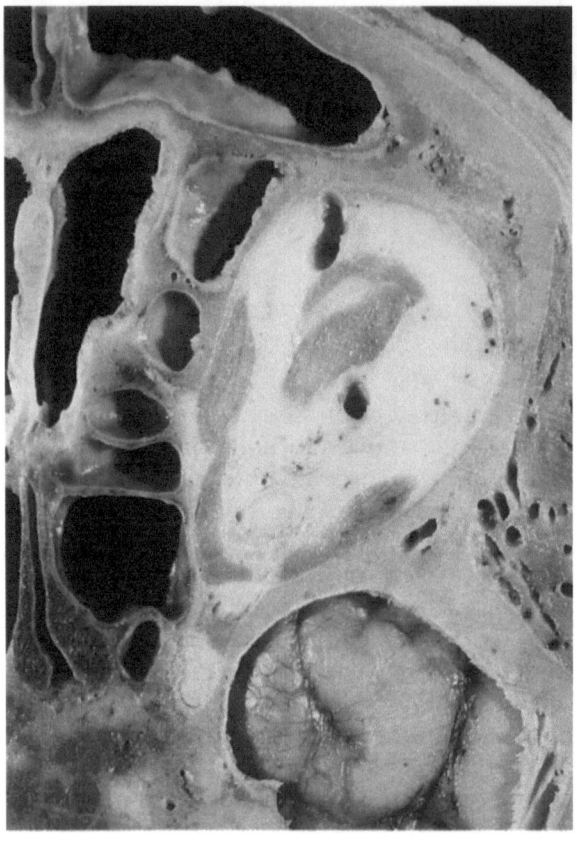

73 b

diagnosis" and order thin-section CT, which can differentiate the four main complications of bacterial sinusitis:

- Septic thrombophlebitis
- Subperiosteal abscess
- Diffuse invasion of septic material into the orbital cavity
- Thrombosis of the cavernous sinus.

Septic Thrombophlebitis

Septic thrombophlebitis is an early orbital complication of bacterial sinusitis. Clinical signs and symptoms include periorbital hyperemia and swelling, ptosis, and proptosis, as well as pain and, occasionally, fever. It is caused by septic material which, due to the increased pressure within the infected sinus, has been pushed into orbital veins draining into the superior ophthalmic vein and into the cavernous sinus. At this stage, CT shows no more than a moderate enlargement of orbital veins and opacification of the adjacent paranasal sinus. All other orbital structures appear normal. At this stage, antibiotic therapy and topical application of a decongestant is all that is needed. Adequate treatment usually results in complete remission with no further complications or residuals.

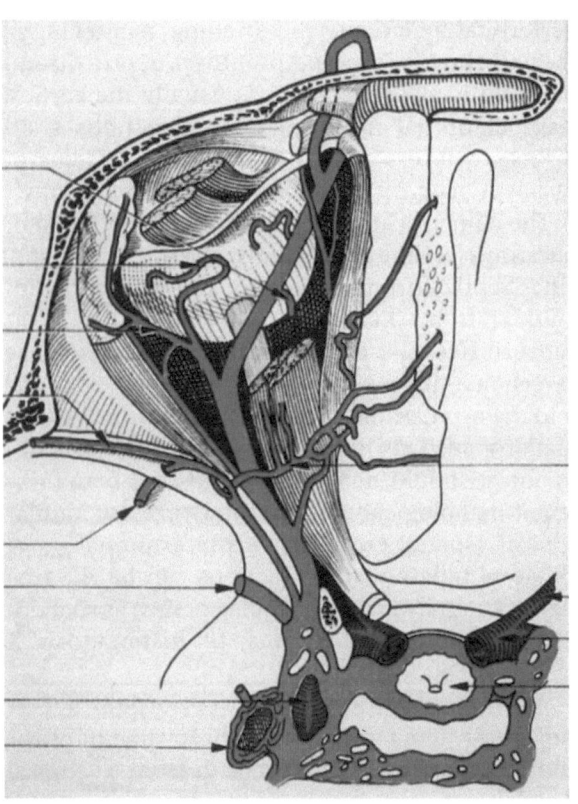

73 c

Figure 73 b, c

b Axial anatomical section through the upper orbit and adjacent ethmoidal air cells.

c Schematic drawing of the venous drainage of ethmoidal air cells and orbital veins. The anterior and posterior ethmoidal air cells drain via the superior ophthalmic veins into the cavernous sinus. Septic material from within the ethmoidal air cells may take this route into the orbital veins and cavernous sinus, causing septic thrombophlebitis or cavernous sinus thrombosis.
(Courtesy of Dr. Jacqueline Vignaud).

Subperiosteal Abscess

Z. T., 1-year-old girl

Once sinus infection has led to bone erosion, septic material from within the sinus is pressed under the periosteum through the bone defect, and a subperiosteal abscess forms. The subperiosteal abscess is clearly delineated against the orbital tissues (Case 74). While antibiotic treatment, if administered promptly, alleviates symptoms and in most cases does lead to a complete remission, there remains a considerable risk for the development of encapsulated abscesses. At times, a change occurs from aerobic to anaerobic organisms which tend to be multiresistant, increasing the danger of cerebral abscesses forming. Therefore, most otorhinolaryngologists continue to consider a subperiosteal abscess an indication for surgical intervention. With regard to the therapeutic approach it is important to differentiate septic thrombophlebitis from a subperiosteal abscess.

History and Clinical Findings
Acute onset of periorbital hyperemia, swelling, and fever.

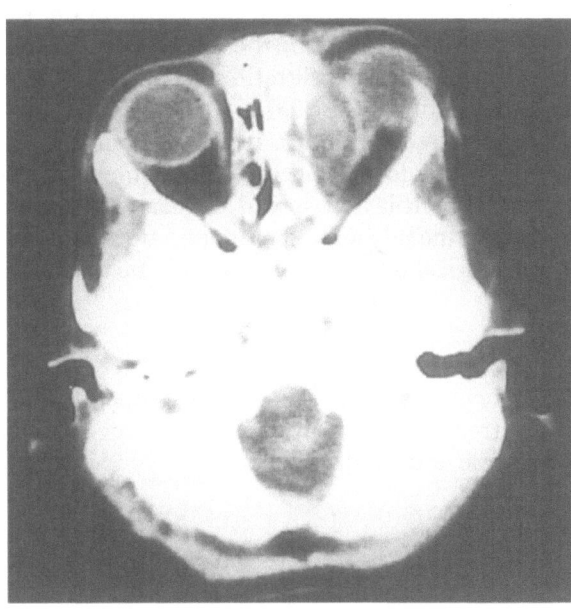

74.1

CT
Unilateral opacification of the upper left ethmoidal air cells. Large soft-tissue area within the medial extraconal space; the mass is sharply demarcated towards the orbital fat. Dislocation of the adjacent extraocular muscle, as well as of the optic nerve and the globe.

Diagnosis
Sinusitis of the ethmoidal air cells and adjacent subperiosteal abscess.

Invasion of Septic Material into the Orbital Cavity

When the periosteum is penetrated, purulent material invades the orbital cavity from the extraconal into the intraconal space. The characteristic CT image shows dense, diffuse infiltration extending continually from the affected sinus into the orbit. The dense infiltration usually masks the orbital structures (Case 75).

Surgical intervention is necessary only in the case of abscess formation. Once septic material has entered the orbit and spread diffusely, antibiotic therapy is the adequate therapeutic option. Additional surgical intervention may only be harmful.

History and Clinical Findings
Upper respiratory tract infection, ineffective antibiotic treatment. Slowly progressive periorbital hyperemia and swelling.

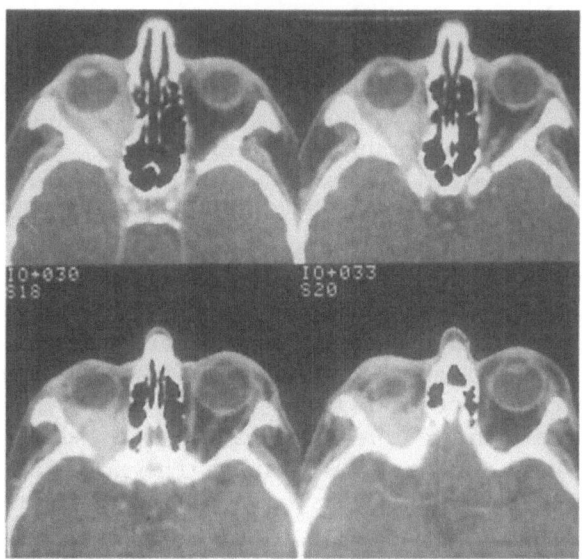

75.2

CT
Opacification of the right maxillary sinus, complete destruction of the orbital floor and diffuse infiltration of the orbital cavity. Downward displacement of the orbital contents.

Diagnosis
Sinusitis of the right maxillary sinus with destruction of the orbital floor and diffuse infiltration of the orbital cavity.

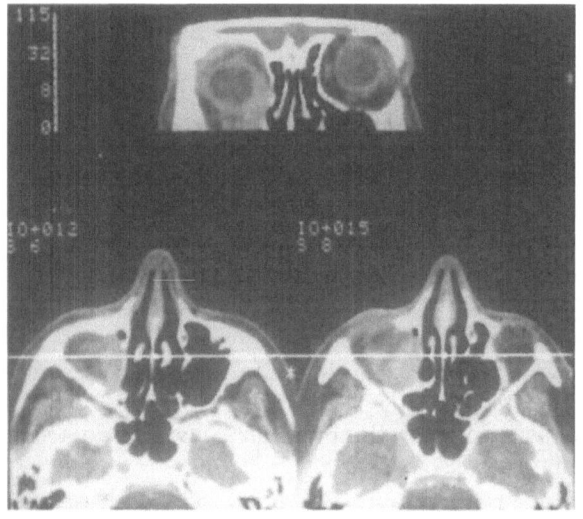

75.1

Septic Thrombosis of the Cavernous Sinus

Spread of septic material from a paranasal sinus via the orbital venous system and superior ophthalmic vein into the cavernous sinus causes septic cavernous sinus thrombosis, which is still a life-threatening situation.

The characteristic CT pattern of cavernous sinus thrombosis consists of an enlargement of the cavernous sinus and massive dilatation of the superior ophthalmic vein, the lumen of which appears dark, indicating the cessation of blood flow consistent with thrombosis (Case 76).

In an early stage a course of intravenous antibiotic treatment is mostly sufficient. Further progression of the thrombosis towards the draining dural sinuses may necessitate systemic anticoagulation, which is associated with a high risk of intracerebral hemorrhage due to the increased intravenous pressure.

60-year-old man

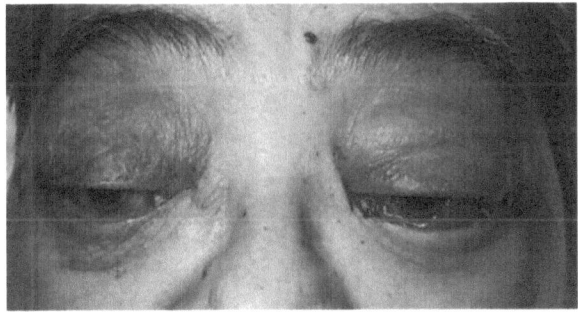

76.1

History and Clinical Findings
Upper respiratory tract infection, fever, bilateral proptosis and chemosis, hyperemia, and periorbital swelling, as well as restricted ocular motility.

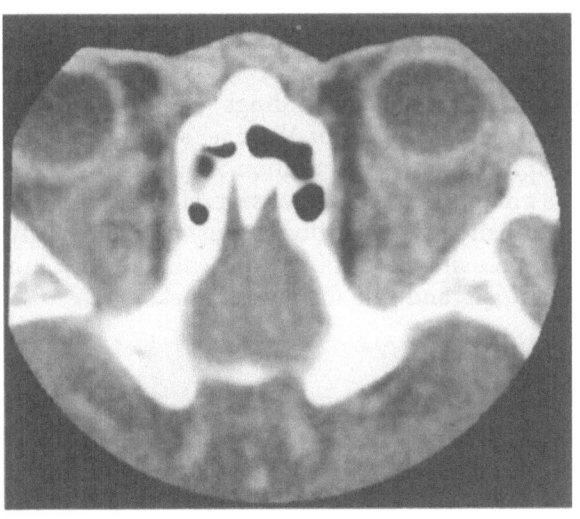

76.2

CT
Massive dilatation of both superior ophthalmic veins, with hypodense lumina, indicating cessation of blood flow consistent with thrombosis.

Diagnosis
Thrombosis of both superior ophthalmic veins and the cavernous sinus.

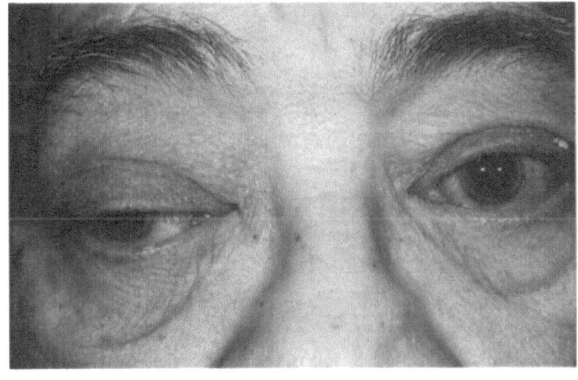

76.3

Clinical Course
Remission of clinical symptomatology after intravenous antibiotic treatment within 24 h (76.3).

Comment
The radiographic findings are pathognomonic.

CT image courtesy of Professor T. H. Newton, former Chief of Neuroradiology, Department of Radiology, University of California Medical School, San Francisco, California, USA.

S. K., 45-year-old woman

History and Clinical Findings
Recurrent episodes of Wegener's granulomatosis
in spite of the administration of cytotoxic substances and corticosteroids for several years (diagnosis
established serologically and histopathologically).

Increasing periorbital hyperemia and swelling,
proptosis, and pain for several weeks.

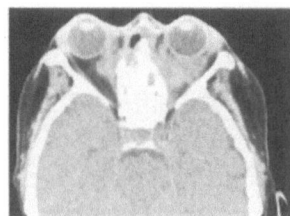

77.1

CT
Opacification of the partially hyperostotic and
partially necrotic ethmoidal air cells with adjacent
soft-tissue masses extending into the orbital cavity.

Diagnosis
Destructive process within the ethmoidal air cells
with orbital soft-tissue masses in a patient with
known Wegener's granulomatosis.

Comment
Had the diagnosis not already been established, a
biopsy would have been required. Differential diagnosis from other necrotizing lesions extending
from the paranasal sinuses into the orbit cannot be
established by radiological means alone.

7 Clinically and Histologically Proven Inflammatory Orbital Diseases and their Differential Diagnoses – Selected on Didactic Grounds

B. I., 60-year-old woman

History and Clinical Findings
Diplopia on right gaze for 4 months.
No pain.

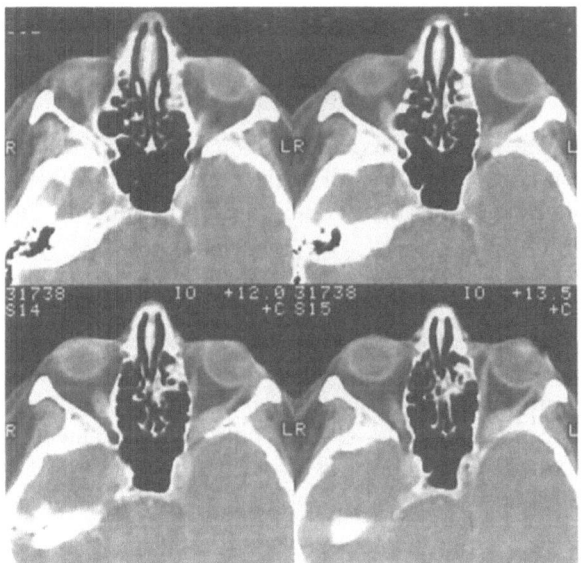

78.1

78.2

CT
Spindle-shaped enlargement of the posterior part of the lateral rectus muscle.

Differential Diagnosis
Most likely a metastasis because of the unusual shape. A search for the underlying malignant neoplasm is necessary.

No pathological findings in chest X-ray, abdominal ultrasound, and bone scintigram.

Cystoscopy
Extended anaplastic carcinoma, originating either in the urinary bladder or the cervix.

Clinical Course
Bilateral hydronephrosis. Pulmonary embolism. Death 6 weeks after diagnosis.

H.M., 63-year-old female

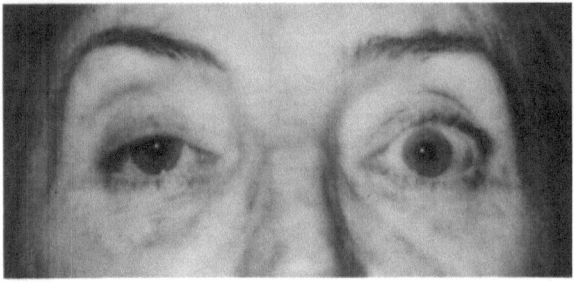

79.1

History and Clinical Findings
Upper respiratory tract infection and right optic
nerve neuritis 3 months ago. Since that time ptosis
of the right eye and hyperemia, diplopia on right
gaze, and enophthalmos of the right eye.

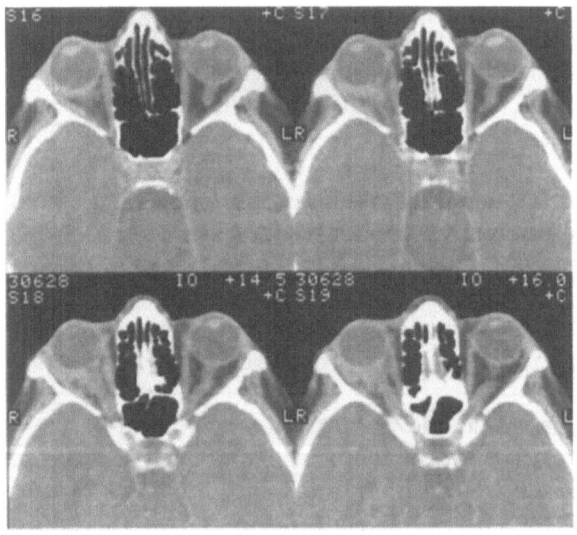

79.2

79.3

CT
In the right intraconal space a large hyperdense
zone encasing the wall of the globe and the extraocular muscles. Lacrimal gland enlargement. Enophthalmos.

Diagnosis
Metastasis of a scirrhous carcinoma of the breast.
Due to the combination of diffuse infiltration and
enophthalmos, a metastasis of a scirrhous carcinoma is most likely. The patient had been diagnosed with scirrhous carcinoma of the breast
years ago.

Comment
In this case, the leading diagnostic elements are the
history and the enophthalmos.

All other inflammatory or neoplastic infiltrations cause proptosis, the exceptions being rare
primary fibrosing and shrinking lesions, as in
idiopathic retroperitoneal fibrosis.

R. J., 5-year-old boy

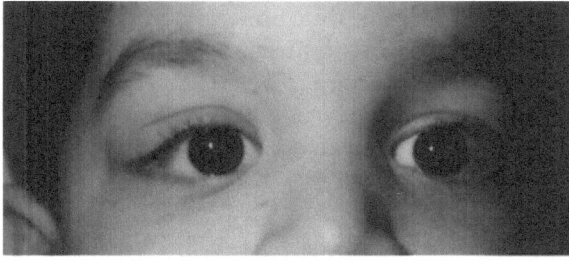

80.1

History and Clinical Findings
Photographs showed that proptosis of the right eye had been existent for several years. This was noticed only after the patient had bumped against the edge of a table.

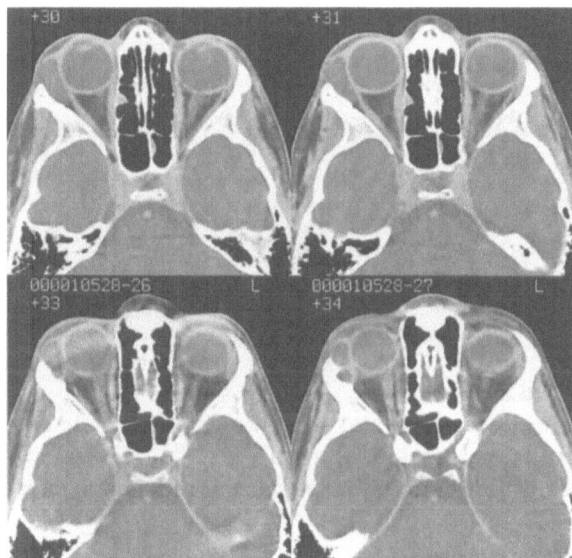

80.2

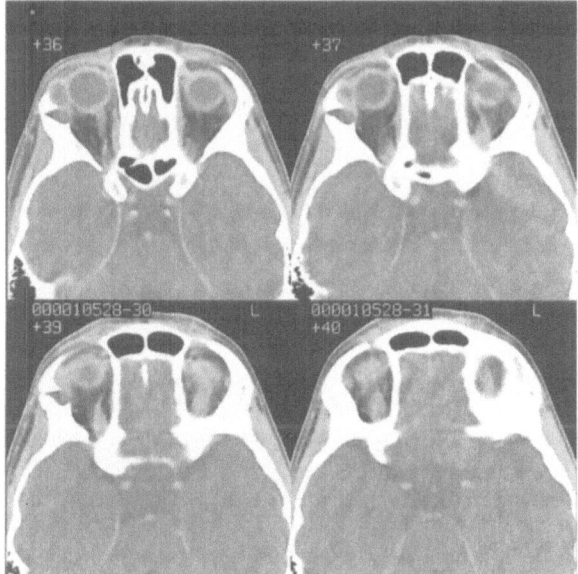

80.3

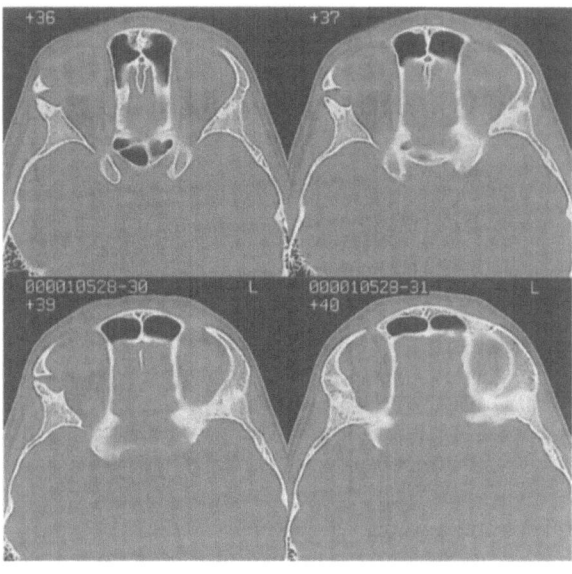

80.4

CT
Compared with the left side, the right orbital wall appears flattened, the bone is focally excavated and in part eroded. Bone defect in the greater wing of the sphenoid bone. The lacrimal gland is displaced superiorly by an oval, smoothly delineated, homogenous, hypodense mass. The globe is indented and displaced medially.

Diagnosis
Dermoid cyst.

Comment
Dermoid cysts tend to rupture, which leads to acute granulomatous inflammatory reactions. Therefore, ruptured dermoid cysts may be mistaken for primary inflammatory or neoplastic lesions of the lacrimal gland. Visualization of the typical bone defect due to longstanding, constant pressure facilitates the diagnosis.

Clinical data courtesy of Professor Hans Borgmann, Department of Ophthalmology, Johanniter Hospital, Bonn, Germany.

M. M., 18-months-old boy

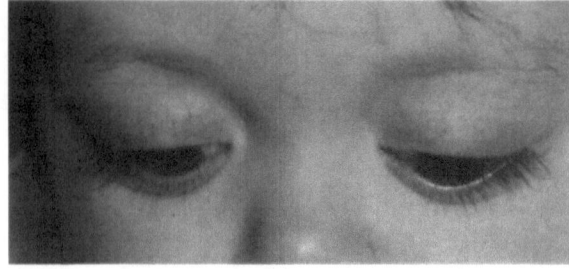

81.1

History and Clinical Findings
Bilateral submandibular lymphadenopathy and recurrent bouts of fever 4 months ago.

Several osteolytic foci in the right scapula and the frontal and parietal skull.

Histopathology (inguinal lymphatic nodes, skin, and tibia biopsies): pathological findings consistent with histiocytosis X.

The patient was presented with subacute onset of proptosis, ptosis, and swelling and hyperemia of both upper lids.

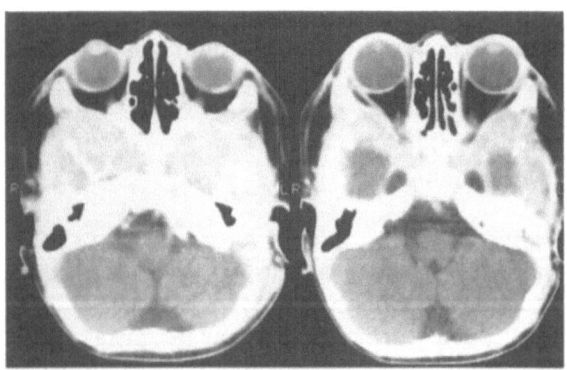

81.2

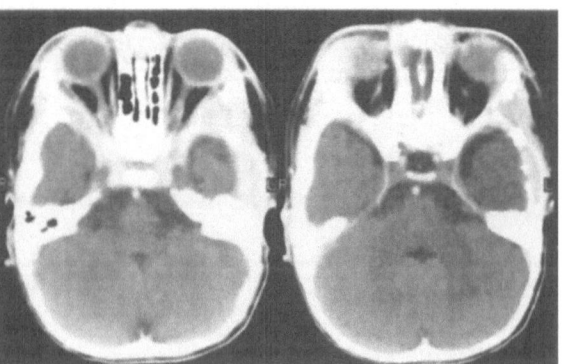

81.3

CT (81.2, 81.3)
Large defects in both greater wings of the sphenoid bone, in the left temporal bone, and in the left orbital roof. Large soft-tissue masses extending into the extradural space.

Dural membrane intact. Adjacent lacrimal glands clearly delineated.

Diagnosis
Histiocytosis X.

Clinical Course
Chemotherapy, followed by remission of clinical signs and symptoms.

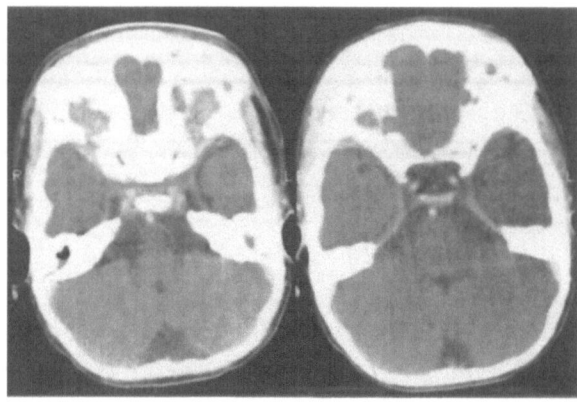

81.4

CT (81.4)
Fifteen months later: Soft-tissue masses in both extraconal spaces. Compared with the previous scans the intracranial lesions are reduced in size.

K. A., 16-year-old girl

History and Clinical Findings
Painful swelling of the left eye, pain increasing with eye movements, for 2 weeks. Local and systemic antibiotic treatment had been ineffective. Considerable chemosis and swelling of the temporal part of the lid. Increasing venous dilatation and incipient papilledema.

Antinuclear antibodies and erythrocyte sedimentation rate elevated.

CT
Moderate enlargement of the left lacrimal gland and enlargement of the peribulbar connective tissue, including Tenon's capsule and the tendons of the rectus muscles.

Diagnosis
Scleritic-tenonitic form of inflammatory orbital pseudotumor with accompanying dacryoadenitis.

Clinical Course
Complete remission of clinical signs and symptoms after steroid treatment.

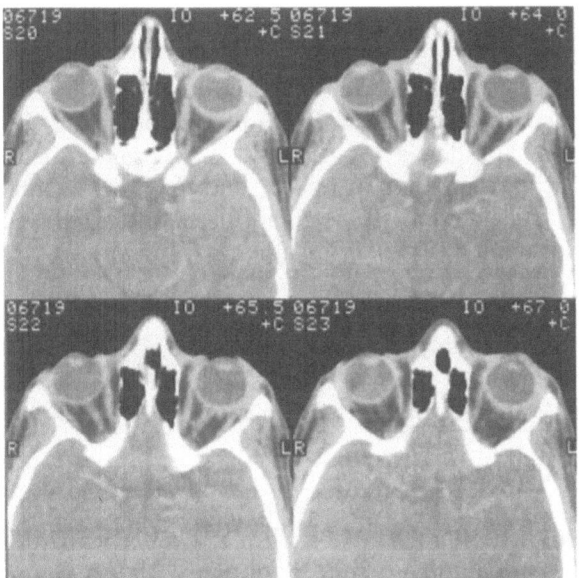
82.1

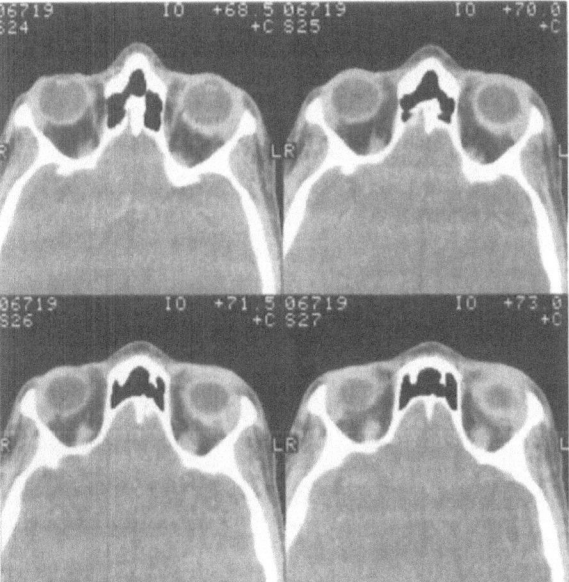
82.2

E. J., 73-year-old man

History and Clinical Findings
Diplopia and generalized restriction of ocular motility. Proptosis and downward displacement of the left globe for 3 weeks.

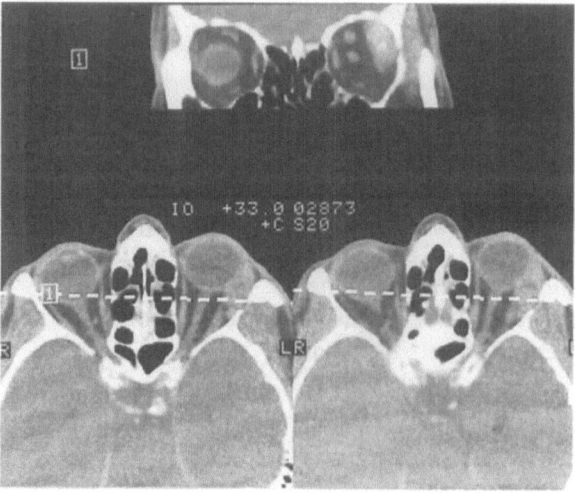

83.3

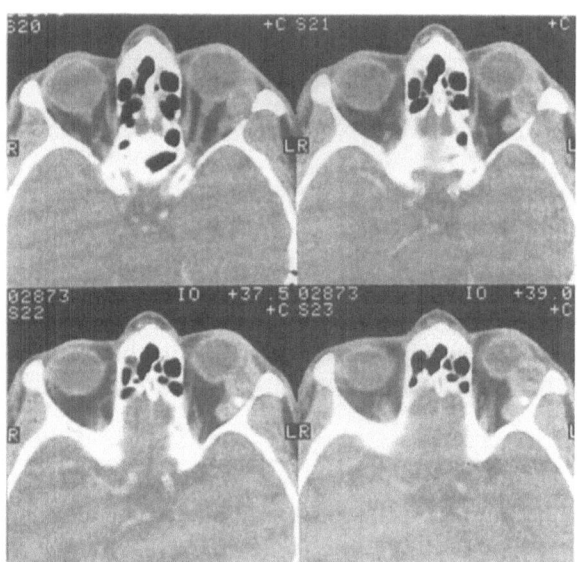

83.1

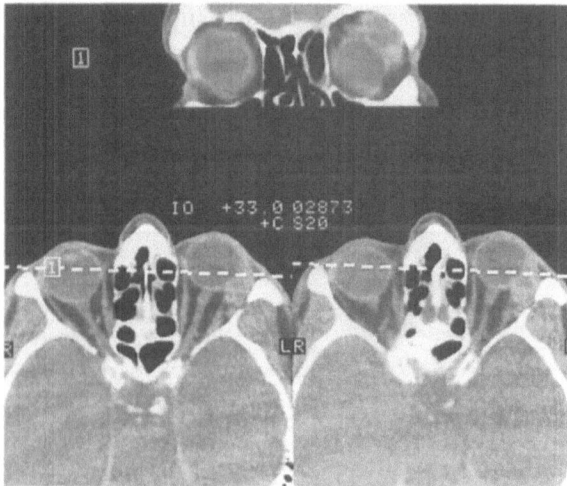

83.2

CT
Large, polycyclic, space-occupying lesion in the area of the left lacrimal gland. Hypodense areas with hyperdense margins, and small punctate calcifications within the mass, and thinning of the adjacent bone. Displacement of the globe and of extraocular muscles. The globe is focally indented.

Differential Diagnosis
Most probably a mixed tumor of the lacrimal gland.

Malignant transformation cannot be excluded.

Clinical Course
An en-bloc resection, leaving the capsule intact and including the adjacent bone, was performed.

Histopathology: mixed tumor of the lacrimal gland (pleomorphic adenoma).

Comment
Bone erosion is supportive of the diagnosis of a slowly growing tumor rather than a mitigated form of abscess-forming dacryoadenitis.

D. H.-G., 60-year-old man

History and Clinical Findings
Painful ophthalmoplegia, Tolosa-Hunt syndrome suspected.

Known sqamous cell carcinoma of the lung (confirmed by biopsy).

Corrected vision 30/100 in each eye. Bilateral central scotomas, more extended on the left side. Third and fourth nerve palsy.

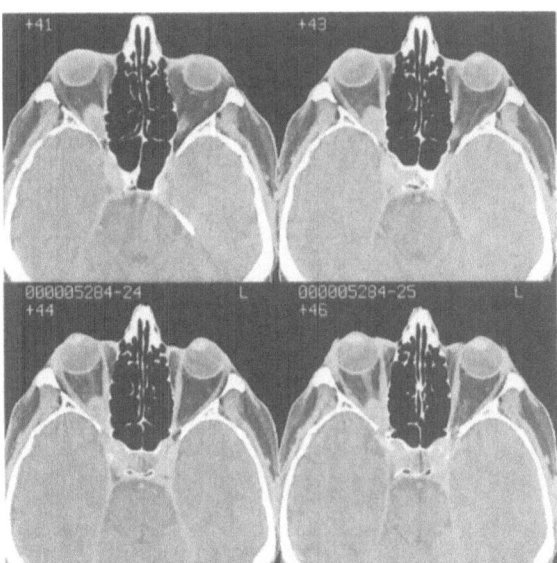

84.1

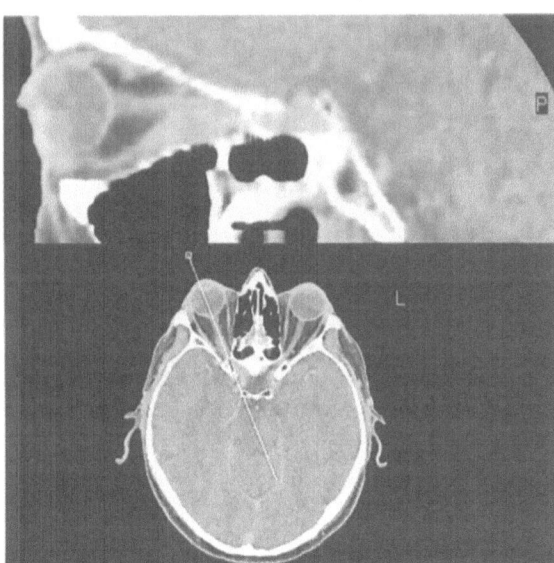

84.2

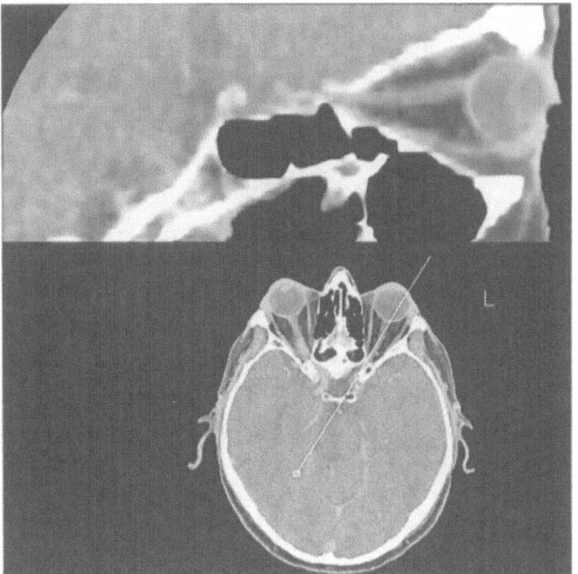

84.3

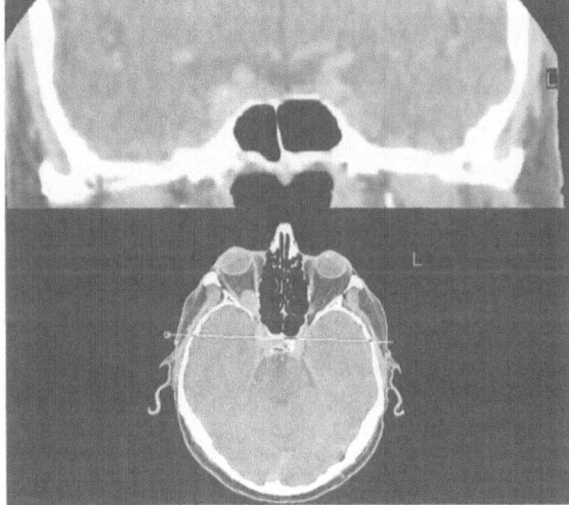

84.4

CT (84.1 – 84.4)
Enlargement of the posterior part of the inferior rectus muscle. Soft-tissue mass, extending through the superior orbital fissure into the right cavernous sinus.

Diagnosis
Metastasis of the squamous cell carcinoma.

Comment
The history of squamous cell carcinoma and the extension of the soft-tissue mass into the cavernous sinus favor the diagnosis of a metastasis.

(Continued on p. 122)

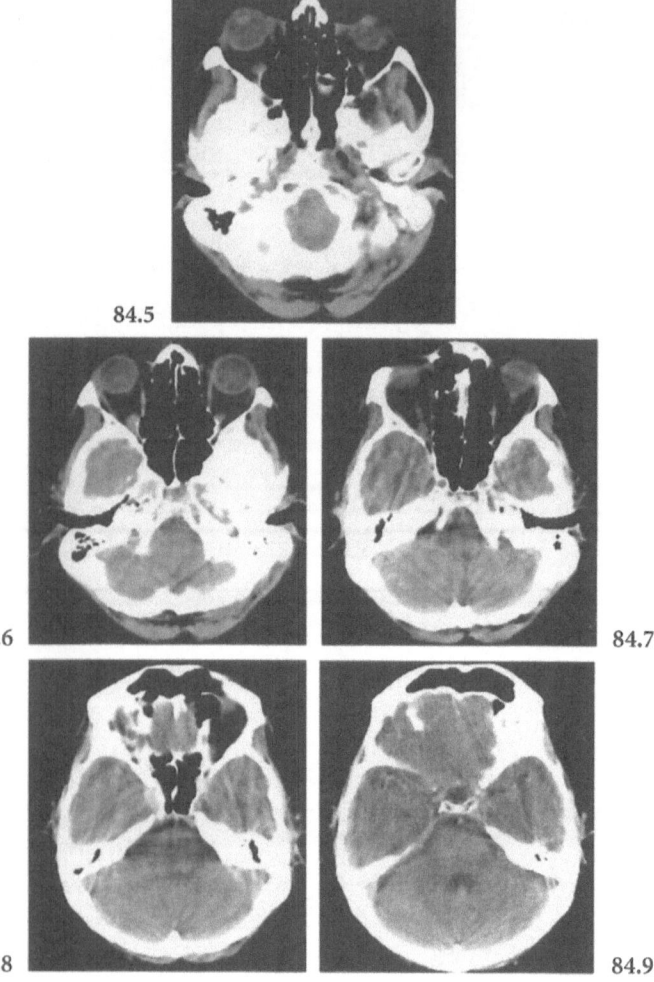

84.5

84.6

84.7

84.8

84.9

CT (84.5 – 84.9)
These CT scans were obtained elsewhere 30 days before the thin-section CT scans (84.1 – 84.4). Section thickness 9 mm, positive angulation approximately 20° to the orbitomeatal baseline. With scans done in this technique, pathological findings may easily be overlooked.

Clinical Course
Radiation therapy.

H. W., 5-year-old boy

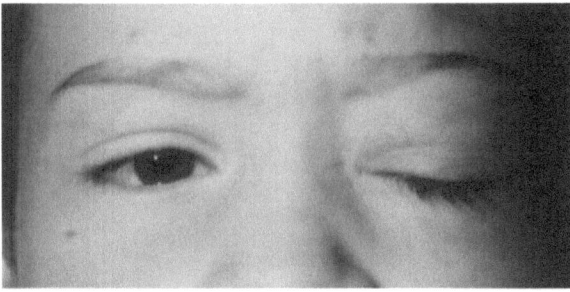

85.1

History and Clinical Findings
Coughing, abdominal pain, and temperature elevated to 102.2 °F (39 °C) 1 week ago. Treatment with penicillin for presumed streptococcal pharyngitis. Admission to hospital the following day due to considerable increase in lid swelling, severe pain and discomfort.

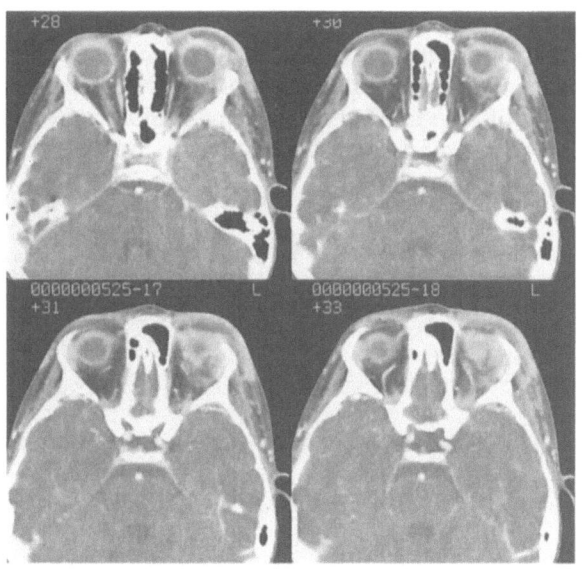

85.3

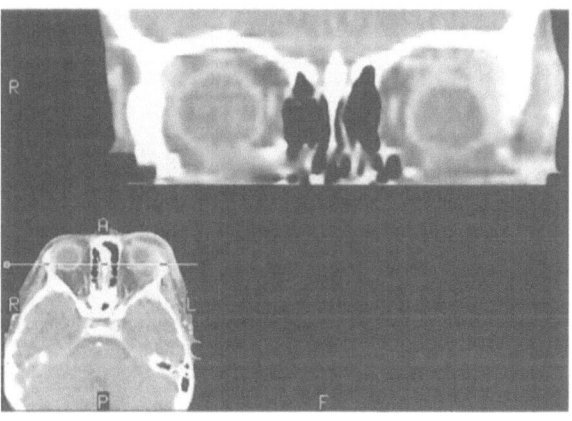

85.4

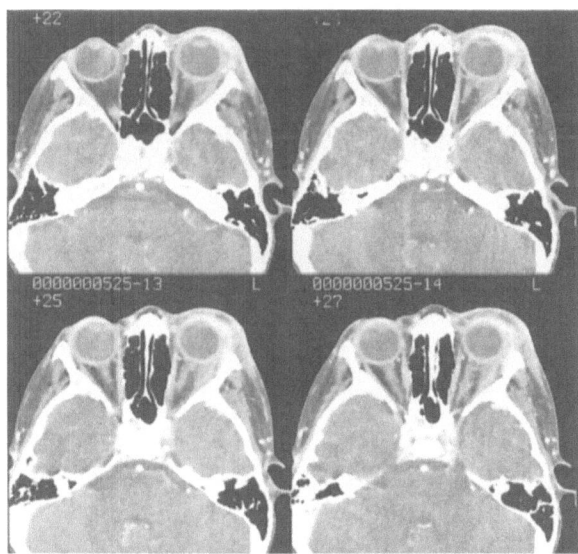

85.2

CT (85.2 – 85.4)
Considerable swelling in the region of the right lateral upper lid. Extended hyperdense areas within the anterior intraconal and extraconal space. Enlargement of the lacrimal gland. Protrusion of the globe. Paranasal sinuses not involved.

Diagnosis
Orbital cellulitis.

(Continued on p. 124)

Clinical Course

Staphylococcus aureus was isolated in the conjunctival smear and a small chalazion was detected.

Significant clinical improvement after a 15-day course of broad-spectrum antibiotics (85.5).

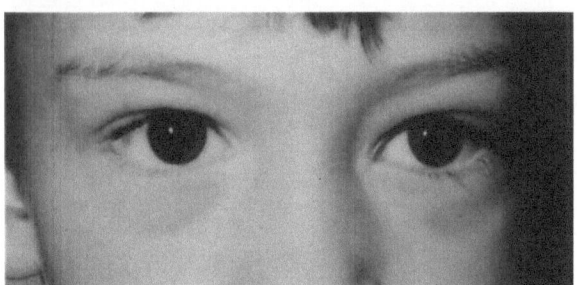

85.5

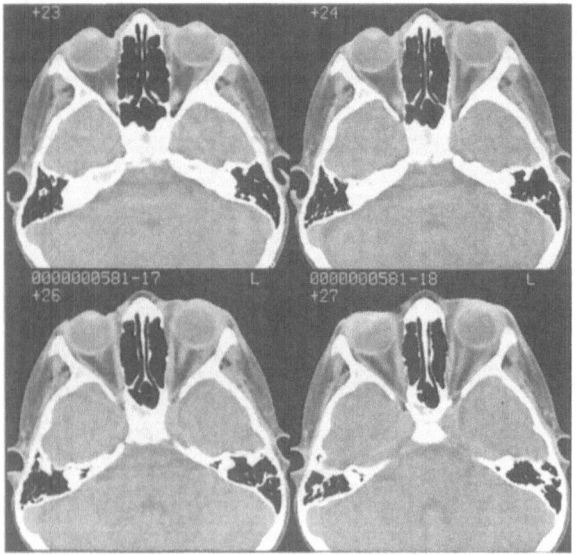

85.6

CT (85.6)
Slight enlargement of the left lid and the lacrimal gland as well as of the lateral rectus muscle.

Diagnosis
Residual inflammatory infiltration of the lids, the lacrimal gland and of the lateral rectus muscle.

Comment
Small children tend to develop secondary infections due to bacterial dissemination which may originate from a small focus that frequently goes unnoticed. The secondary infection may develop in an area not necessarily close to the original focus.

N. H., 52-year-old woman

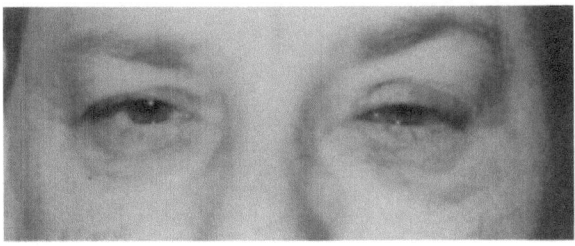

86.1

History and Clinical Findings
Sensation of burning and pain in the left eye, as well as blurred vision, for the past 3 months. Recurrence of symptoms after discontinuation of steroid treatment.

Swelling of the temporal part of the left upper lid. Periorbital swelling and chemosis.

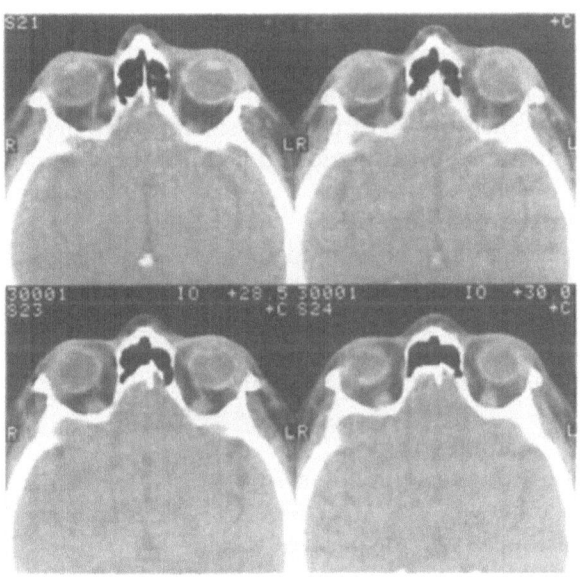

86.2

CT
Unilateral swelling of the left upper lid, moderate enlargement of the lacrimal gland, and slight enlargement and contrast enhancement of the wall of the left globe.

Diagnosis
Dacryoadenitic form of inflammatory orbital pseudotumor.

S. H.-J., 37-year-old man

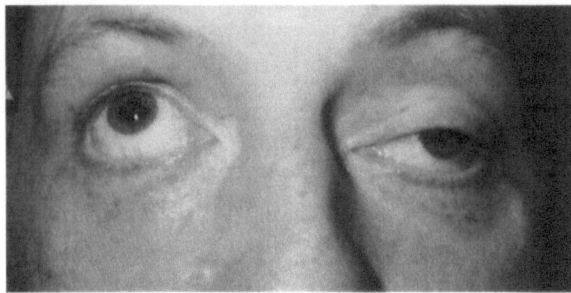

87.1

Attempted upward gaze

History and Clinical Findings
Acute onset of ptosis 3 weeks ago, limitation of upward gaze, severe pain in the left eye and diplopia.
    Pituitary gland adenoma? Hypophyseal tumor? Tolosa-Hunt syndrome? Aneurysm?

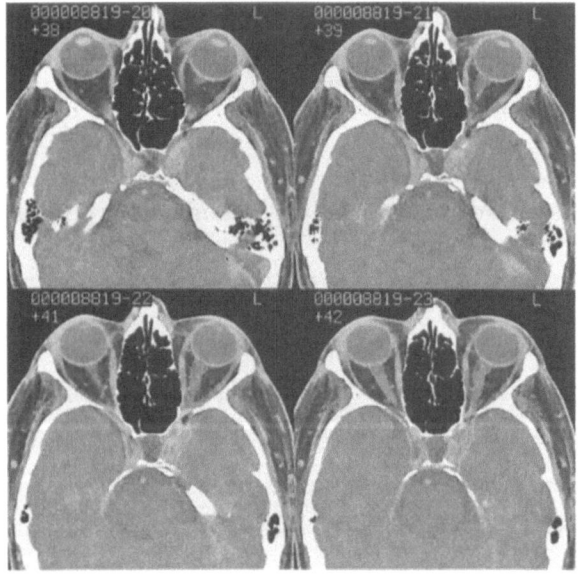

87.2

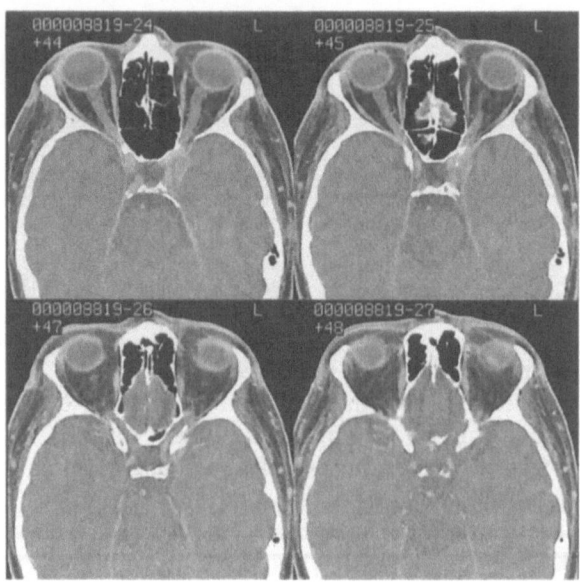

87.3

CT
Enlargement of the left cavernous sinus, its lateral wall protruding. The adjacent clinoid process appears surrounded by a soft-tissue mass. No hyperostosis of adjacent bone and no focal "blistering".

Differential Diagnosis
Diagnosis cannot be made by radiological means alone. Because of the absence of hyperostosis, however, a meningioma is not likely. A flat soft-tissue mass surrounding the anterior clinoid process indicates an aneurysm is also highly unlikely.

Histopathology
Non-Hodgkin lymphoma. HIV infection, previously unknown, was ascertained. Other lymphomas were located in the paravertebral region.

L. F., 53-year-old man

History and Clinical Findings
Progressive somnolence, mydriasis, pupillary reaction absent.

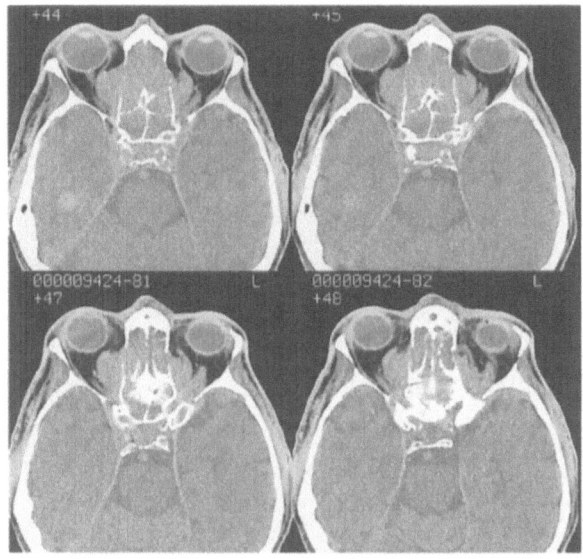

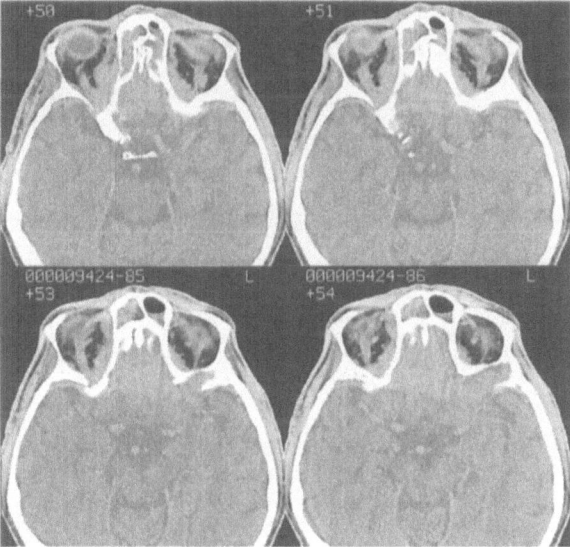

38.1

8.2

CT
Large space-occupying lesion within the ethmoidal air cells and the sphenoid sinuses, extending into both extraconal spaces. Displacement of both medial rectus muscles. Compression of the optic nerve within the orbital apex.

The tumor also extends into the cavernous sinus and into the intracranial space. Destruction of the lamina cribrosa. Butterfly-shaped extension of the tumor into the anterior cranial fossa. Inferiorly extension of the tumor into the nasal cavities.

Differential Diagnosis
Destructive lesion, most probably originating in the ethmoidal air cells, such as an esthesioneuroblastoma, or a destructive granulomatous lesion, such as in Wegener's granulomatosis or midline granuloma.

Histopathology
Poorly differentiated nonkeratinizing squamous cell carcinoma, WHO grade III.

S. P., 71-year-old man

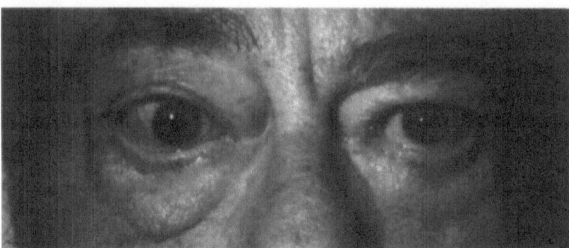

89.1

History and Clinical Findings

Graves' disease was diagnosed 6 years ago. Therapy with radioiodine 2 years ago was followed by increasing proptosis of the right eye. Progressive visual loss and visual field defects as well as diplopia.

Combined treatment with steroids and radiation was followed by remission of proptosis; visual loss and diplopia, however, increased.

No change in CT findings which could explain the progressive visual loss.

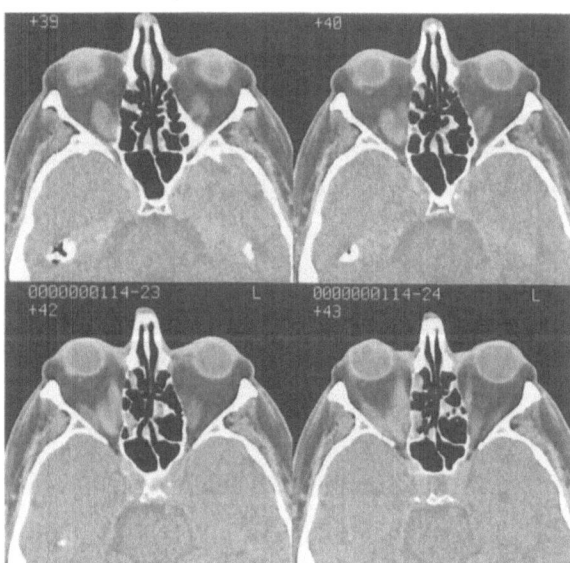

89.2

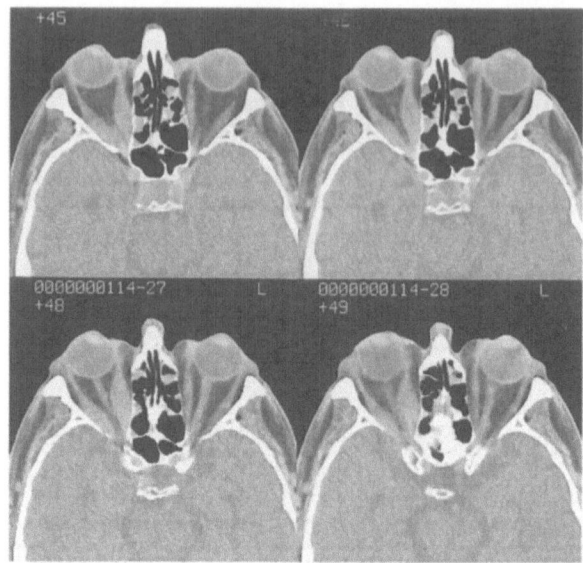

89.3

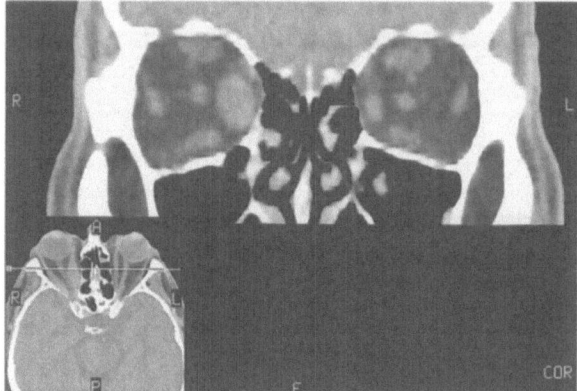

89.4

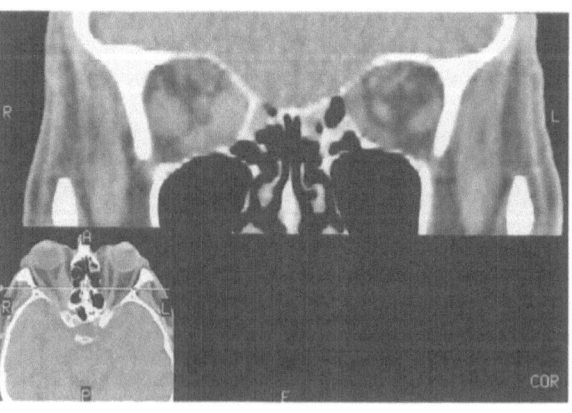

89.5

(Continued on p. 129)

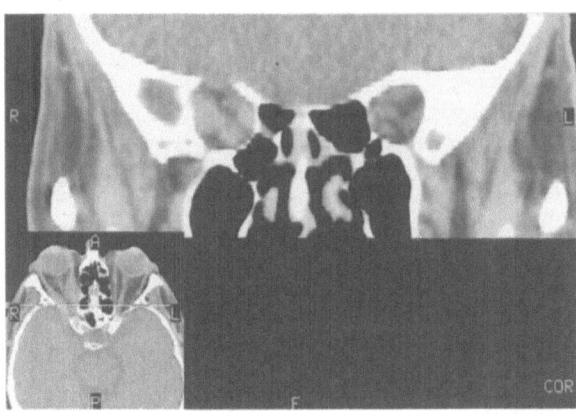

89.6

CT

Enlargement of most extraocular muscles on the right side and of the superior rectus muscle on the left side. Areas of lower density within both superior rectus muscles. Erosion of the right orbital roof.

Diagnosis

Bilateral polymyositic form of Graves' disease, with fibrotic changes, more pronounced on the right side. Spontaneous decompression.

Comment

Progressive visual loss and visual field defects were caused by cardiogenic embolism due to atrial fibrillation. Systemic anticoagulation with warfarin resulted in both improvement of visual acuity (right eye: from 20/100 to 70/100), and gradual remission of visual field defects.

Radiation of the orbital apex was repeated and resulted in remission of proptosis.

J.E., 31-year-old woman

History and Clinical Findings
Severe pain behind the eye, proptosis and peri-orbital hyperemia, for 1 week. Visual loss in the right eye for 3 days.

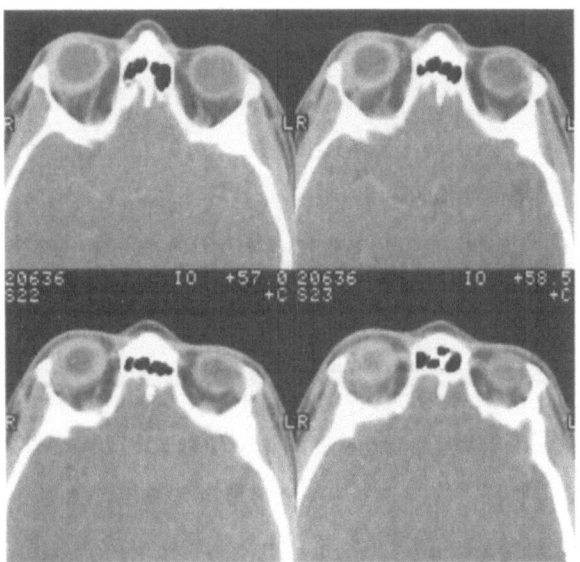

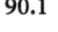
90.1

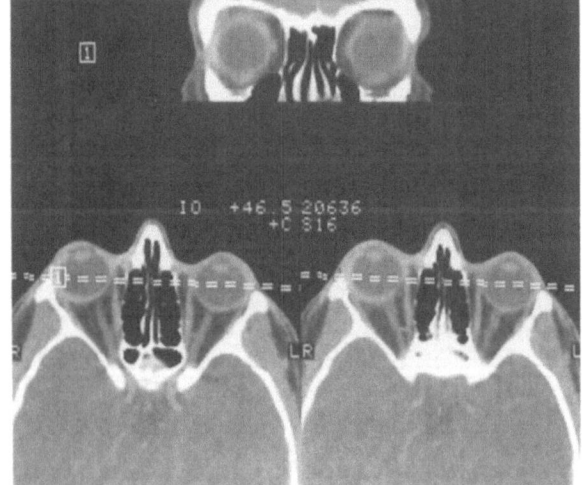
90.2

CT
Considerable enlargement of the wall of the right globe and of the lacrimal gland.

Diagnosis
Scleritic-tenonitic form of inflammatory orbital pseudotumor with involvement of the lacrimal gland.

Clinical Course
Complete remission of clinical signs and symptoms and of pathological CT findings following steroid treatment (beginning with 100 mg prednisolone, gradually reducing the dose).

R.R., 44-year-old woman

History and Clinical Findings
Hyperlacrimation and blurred vision in the right eye, severe photophobia, diplopia and pain for 3 weeks. Palsy of the right abducent nerve. No pathological findings in the cerebrospinal fluid.

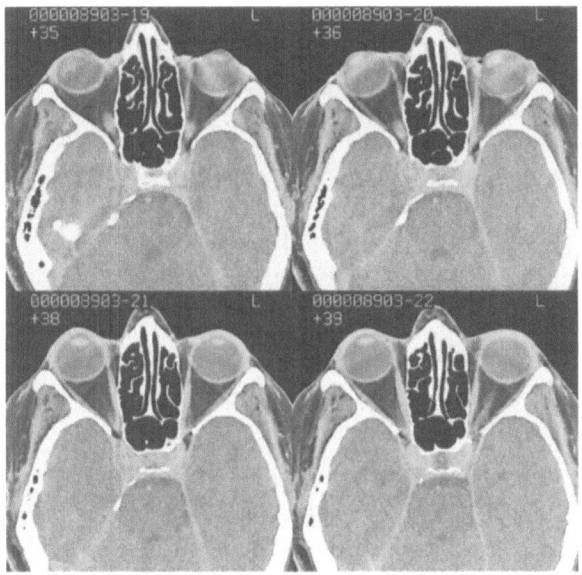

91.1

CT
Considerable enlargement of the right cavernous sinus by a roundish, space-occupying, contrast-enhancing lesion. The dural membrane is displaced laterally, the carotid artery medially.

Symptoms responded impressively to steroid treatment. The clear delineation of the lesion, however, is evidence against inflammatory or neoplastic infiltration.

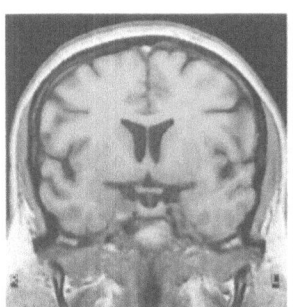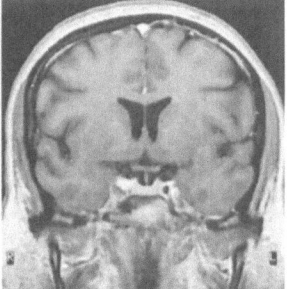

2–3

MRI (91.2, 91.3)
Well-defined, roundish lesion of low signal intensity and intense contrast enhancement within the cavernous sinus.

Angiography should be performed to exclude thrombosis within the aneurysm as well as a meningioma.

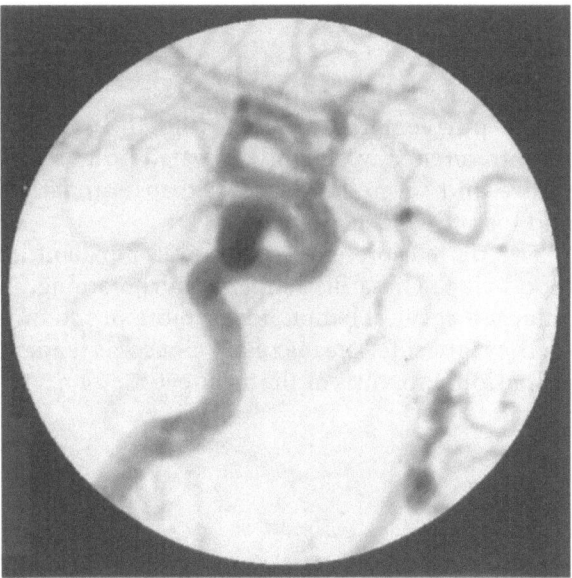

91.4

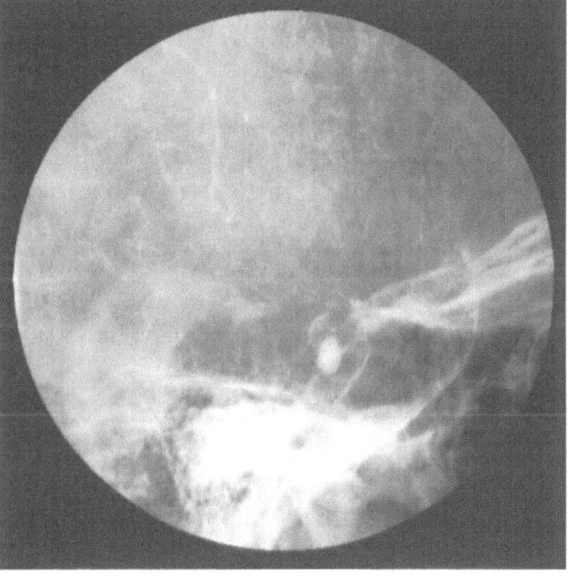

91.5

Angiography (91.4, 91.5)
Pedunculated carotid artery aneurysm within the cavernous sinus.

Therapy
Coil occlusion.

Angiograms courtesy of Dr. Nilson, Chief of Department of Radiology, German Red Cross Hospital, Neuwied, Germany.

M. O., 7-year-old boy

H. E., 75-year-old man

History and Clinical Findings
Acute purulent rhinitis for a month. Antibiotic therapy ineffective. Slightly elevated body temperature and severe headaches, exhaustion, fatigue, and loss of weight.

The patient presented with fever, purulent and blood-tinged nasal discharge, mouth breathing, and enlarged cervical lymph nodes, more pronounced on the right side. The maxillary sinus was tender to palpation. Proptosis of the right eye for 24 h.

History and Clinical Findings
Increasing proptosis and lateral deviation of the globe for the past few months. Restricted adduction, diplopia, chemosis, and orbital pain. No improvement with steroid treatment.

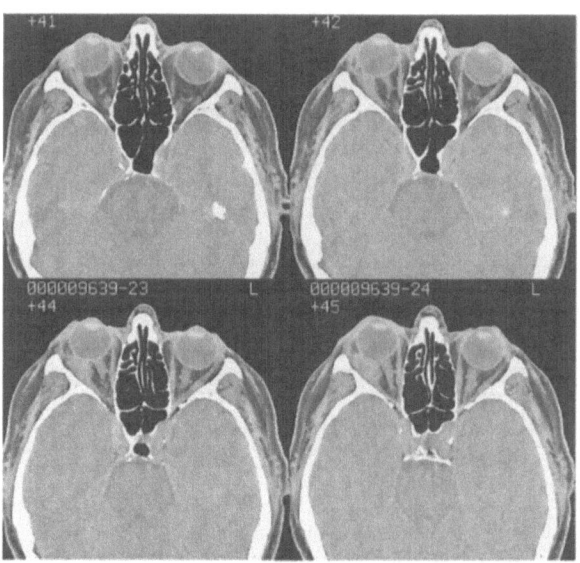

93.1

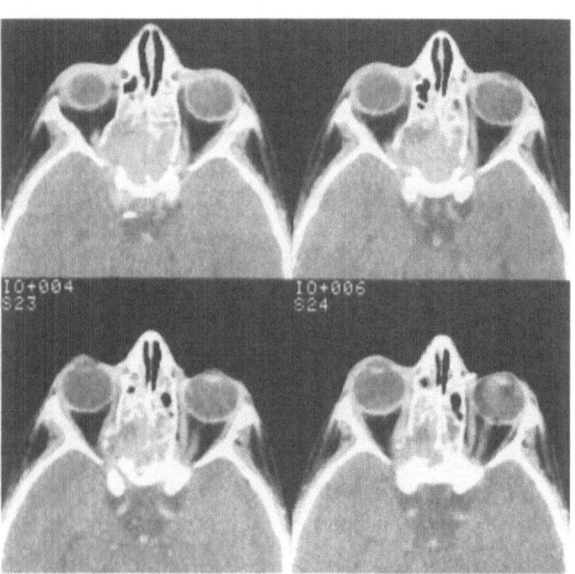

92.1

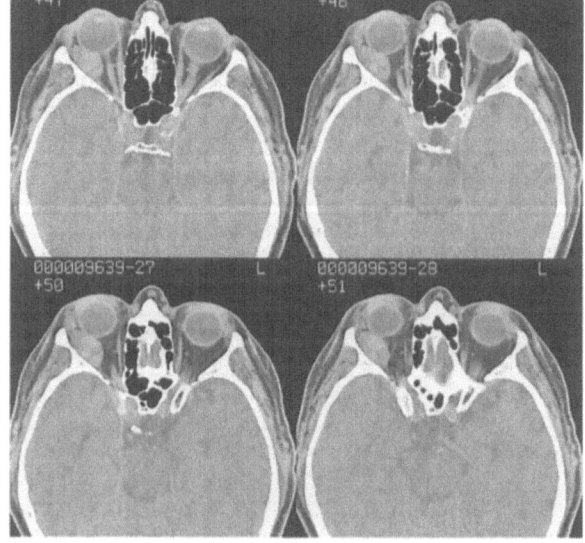

93.2

CT
Large, destructive, solid, space-occupying lesion in both nasal cavities, ethmoidal air cells and sphenoid sinuses. The mass invades the maxillary sinuses and the orbits, more extensively on the right side. The tumor also invades the anterior cranial fossa and the cavernous sinus and destroys the floor of the sella turcica. Bilaterally, destruction of the lesser wing of the sphenoid bone.

Differential Diagnosis
Considering the patient's age, rhabdomyosarcoma or metastasis of a neuroblastoma are the most likely diagnoses.

Histopathology
Rhabdomyosarcoma.

Therapy
Combined radiation therapy and chemotherapy.

(Continued on p. 133)

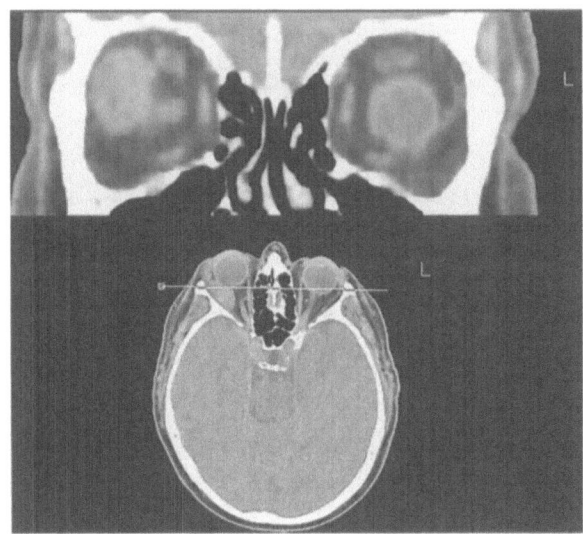

93.3

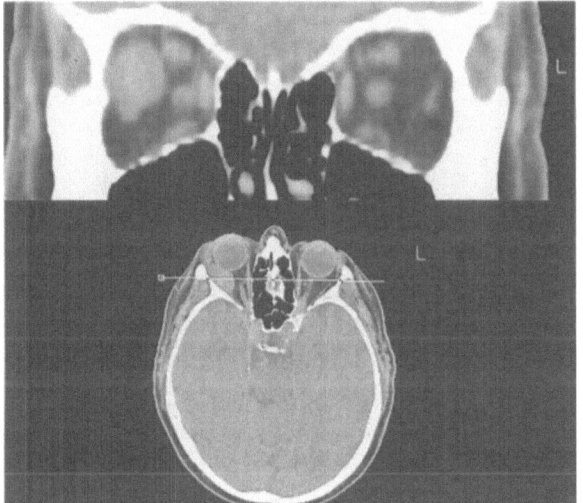

93.4

CT
Large, homogeneous, well-defined, space-occupying lesion in the right anterior and superior extraconal space, bordering on the lateral rectus muscle and on the globe. Clear delineation of the lacrimal gland. No destruction of adjacent bone.

Diagnosis
Space-occupying lesion closely related to the right lateral rectus muscle. The nature of the lesion cannot be determined by CT alone. A biopsy is necessary.

Histopathology
Solitary fibroma.

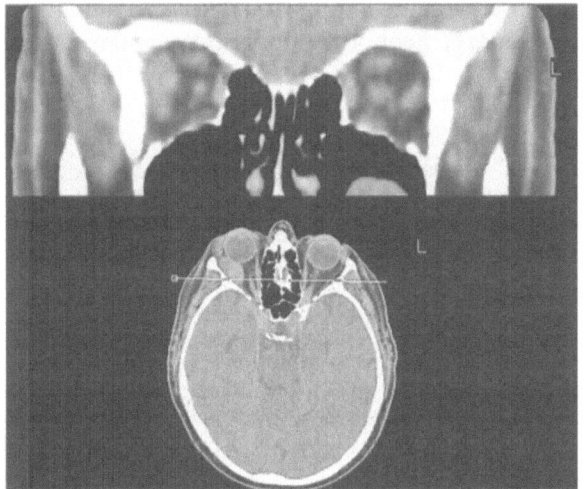

93.5

P. B., 69-year-old man

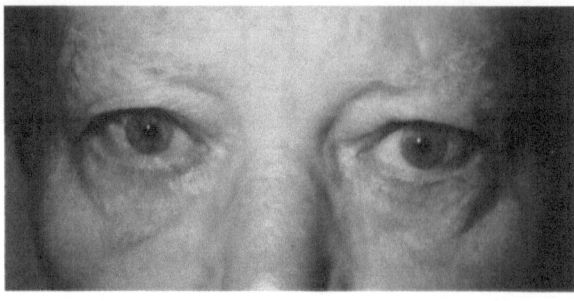

94.1

History and Clinical Findings

Hyperthyroidism was diagnosed 1 year ago. The patient takes antithyroid medication.

Swelling and hyperemia of the lids and sensation of pressure within the orbit for the past 4 months.

Bilateral slight proptosis, chemosis, and temporally accentuated lid swelling.

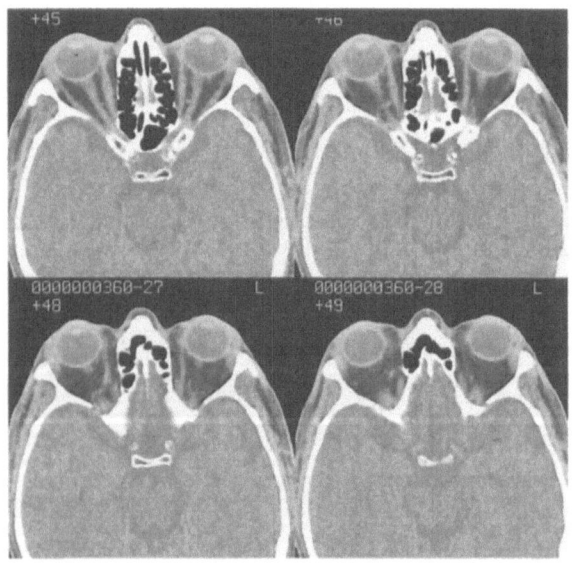

94.2

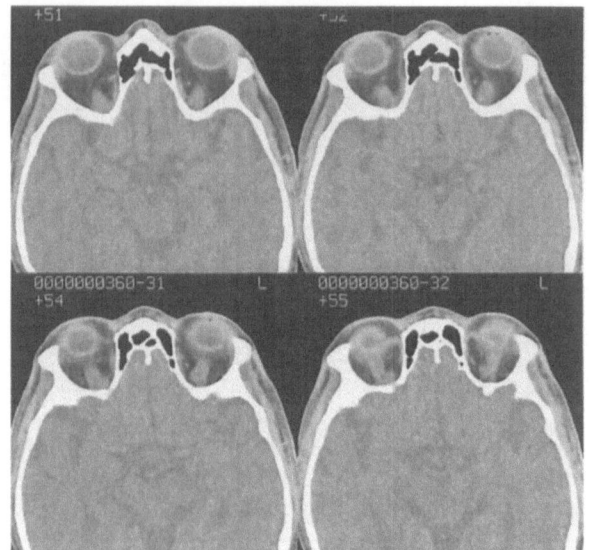

94.3

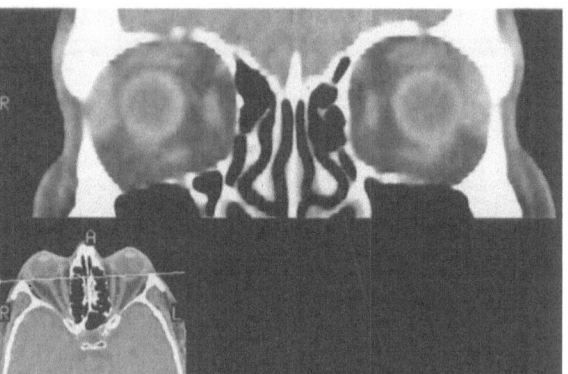

94.4

CT

Bilateral lacrimal gland enlargement, slightly increased volume of the orbital fat, and slight bilateral enlargement of the upper extraocular muscle complex.

Diagnosis

Graves' disease, predominantly dacryoadenitic form.

Radiation therapy scheduled.

T. R., 3-month-old girl

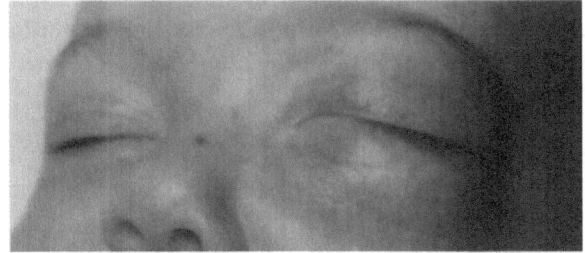

History and Clinical Findings
Hemangiomatous skin lesions in the abdomen and in the toes. Protrusion of the left globe. Livid discoloration of the lids. Capillary hemangioma suspected.

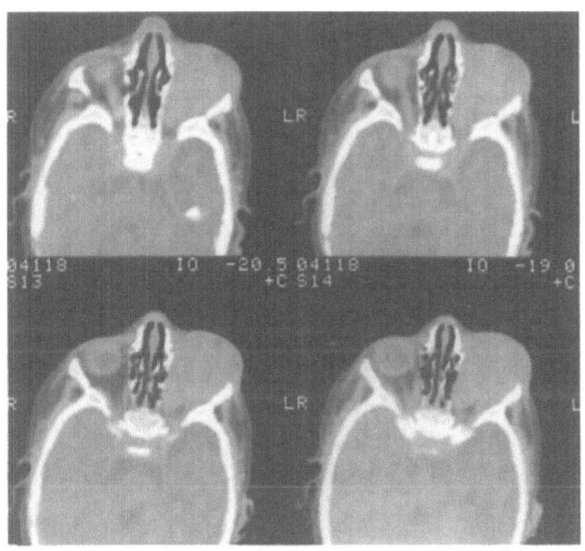

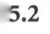

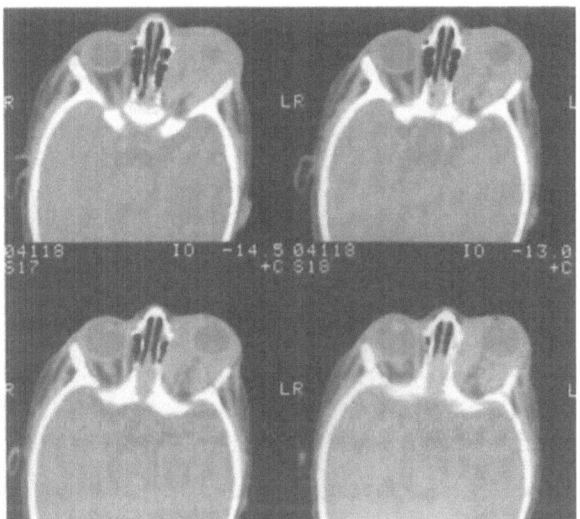

CT
Large soft-tissue masses within the left orbit. Widespread excavation of the bony orbit. Most orbital structures are masked.

Diagnosis
Capillary hemangioma.

Clinical Course
Remission after systemic steroid treatment.

Comment
The excavations of the bony orbit are indicative of a slowly growing tumor. Together with the clinical features, the CT findings allow the diagnosis to be made with a high degree of safety.

H. A., 49-year-old woman

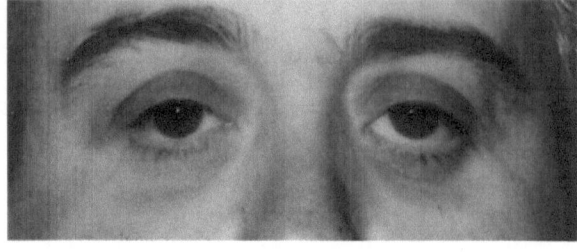

96.1

History and Clinical Findings
Proptosis, sensation of pressure behind the left eye, blurred vision, and restricted ocular motility.

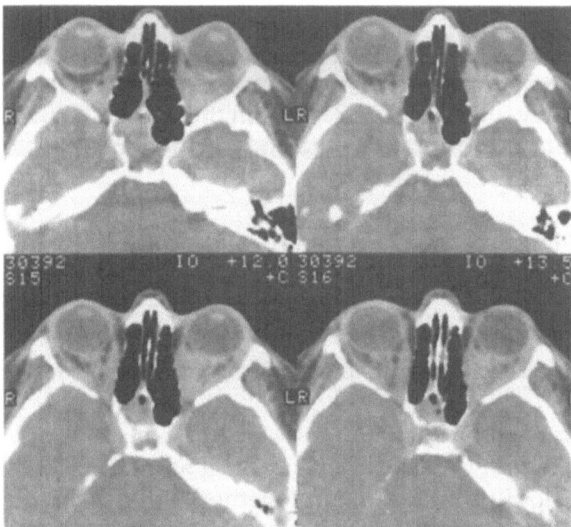

96.2

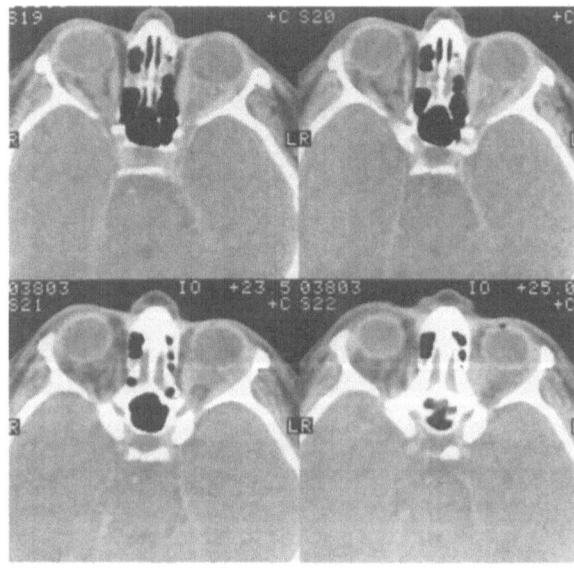

96.3

CT (96.2, 96.3)
Extended hyperdense areas within both orbits. Swelling of the adjacent extraocular muscles. Slight enlargement of the lacrimal gland. Part of the optic nerve appears as a band-shaped area of lower density.

Differential Diagnosis
Diffusely infiltrating form of inflammatory orbital pseudotumor, lymphatic disease, or metastatic infiltration.
　　Further diagnostic tests necessary.

Biopsy (orbit)
Metastasis of a scirrhous carcinoma of the breast.

Clinical Course
The patient was diagnosed with metastasizing cancer of the breast.

Chemotherapy.

96.4

CT (96.4)
Two years later: Almost identical findings. In spite of extended diffuse infiltration, no protrusion of the globe.

Comment
The absence of exophthalmos despite extended diffuse orbital infiltration is suggestive of a metastasis of a scirrhous carcinoma.

T. B., 77-year-old man

History and Clinical Findings

Recurrent fistulas and abscesses above the left maxilla for the past 10 years.

Last year, the patient was hospitalized due to a suspected carcinoma within the maxilla. Complaints of pain on the left side of his face radiating to the ear.

Skull X-ray: destruction of the left upper alveolar process with opacification of the complete left maxillary sinus, the medial wall of which cannot be clearly delineated.

Surgical biopsies from the alveolar process and the hard palate: granulomatous inflammatory process with papillar epithelial hyperplasia and cell dysplasia. No invasive tumor.

The patient refused the recommended surgery.

At present, considerable swelling and hyperemia of the left cheek and of the lids. Orifice of a fistula above the left zygomatic bone, purulent discharge. Older orifice in the left temple.

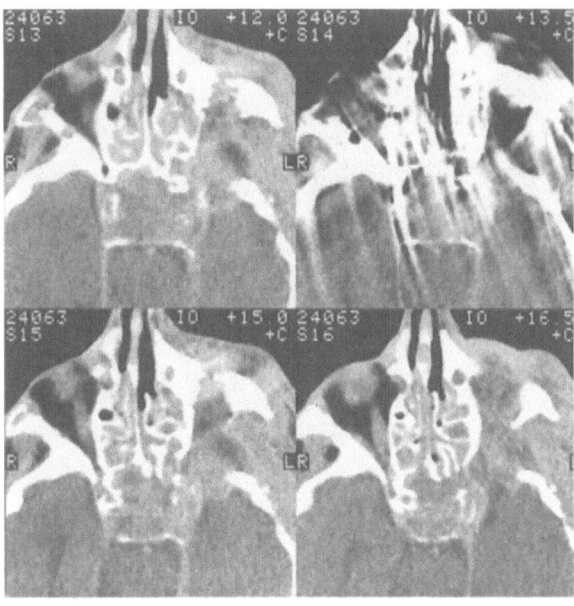

97.2

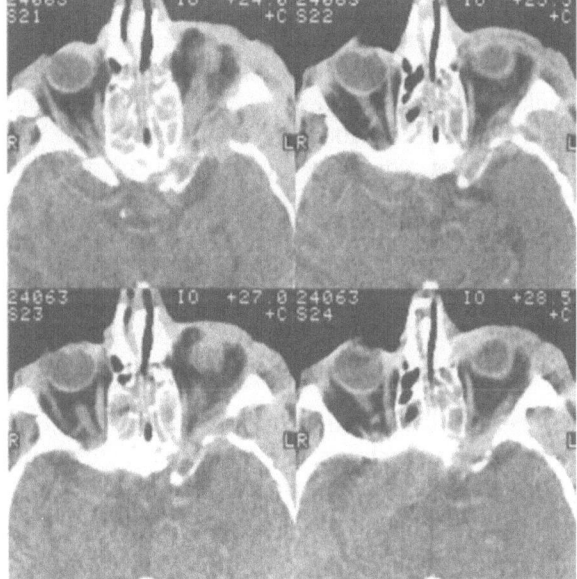

97.3

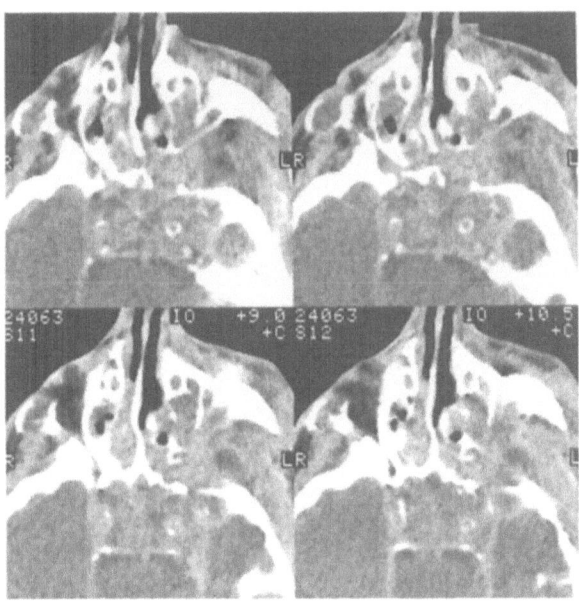

97.1

(Continued on p. 138)

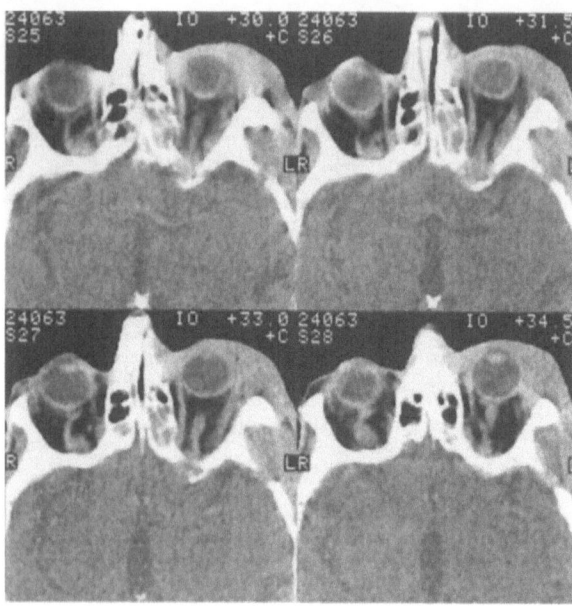

97.4

CT
Large hyperdense areas in both maxillary sinuses, in both the ethmoidal air cells, and within the left cheek and temple. Large bone defects in the maxilla and in the orbits, more pronounced on the left side. Almost complete destruction of the left sphenoidal wing, of the clive, and of the tips of both petrosal bones. Infiltration of the left orbit and of the sella. The cavernous sinus and the internal carotid artery are laterally displaced. Bone defect in the left temporal bone. The dural membrane while displaced appears intact.

Differential Diagnosis
Most likely a slowly-growing, infiltrating, destructive tumor with secondary infection.

Clinical Course
Definite histopathological diagnosis: keratinizing squamous cell carcinoma.
    Radiation therapy.
    Death 4 months later.

Comment
In recurrent infections of the viscerocranium, an underlying neoplasm must be excluded.

S. T., 72-year-old woman

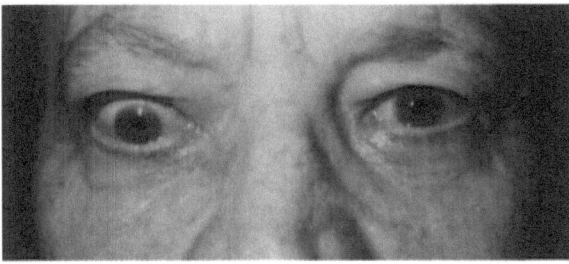

98.1

History and Clinical Findings

Hyperthyroidism was diagnosed 2 years ago, when the patient complained of palpitations. Antithyroid medication.

Onset of Graves' ophthalmopathy 6 weeks later.

Presently, proptosis and lid retraction as well as restricted ocular motility and diplopia.

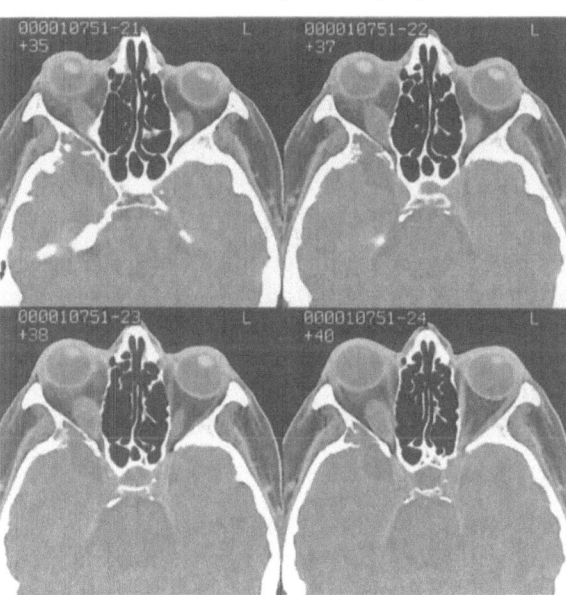

98.2

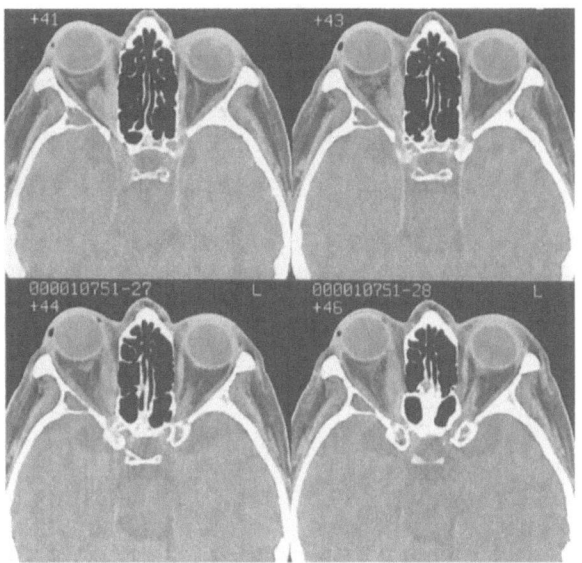

98.3

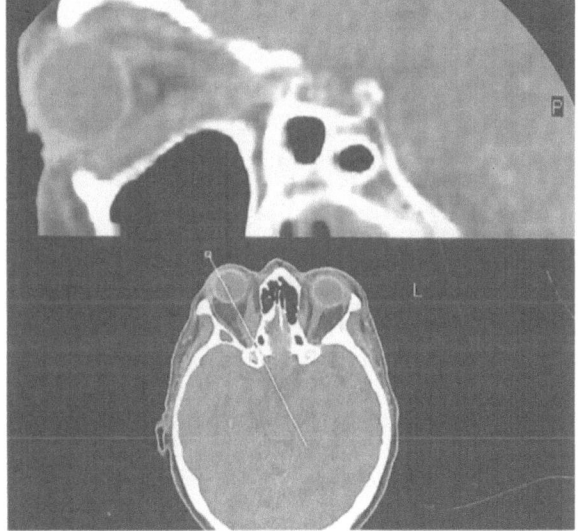

98.4

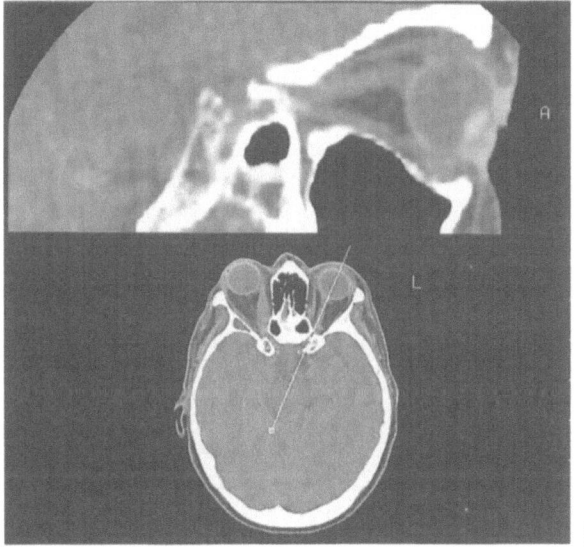

98.5

(Continued on p. 140)

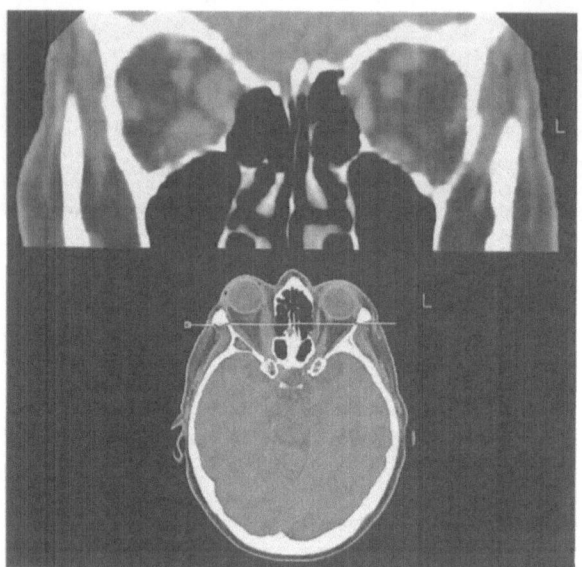

98.6

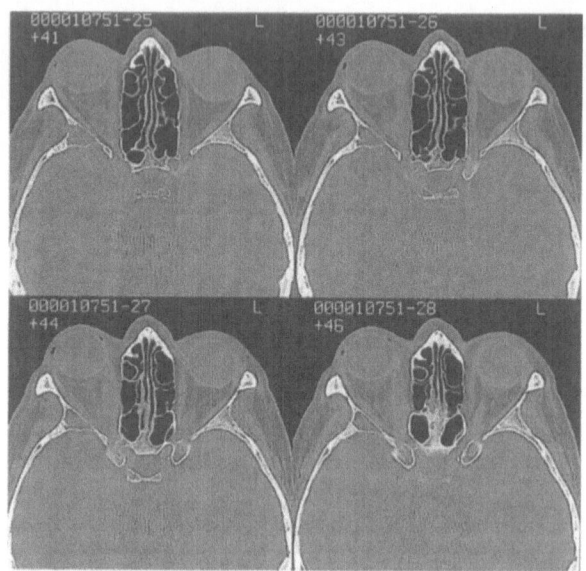

98.9

CT
Unilateral enlargement of several extraocular muscles. Protrusion of the globe. Areas of lower density within several extraocular muscles indicate fibrotic transformation.

Incidental Findings
Within the right sphenoid wing, part of the spongiosa is replaced by soft tissue; the dorsal cortical substance is in part eroded. Most likely diagnosis: intraosseous dermoid.

Diagnosis
Unilateral, polymyositic form of Graves' disease.

Clinical Course
Spontaneous remission of symptoms.

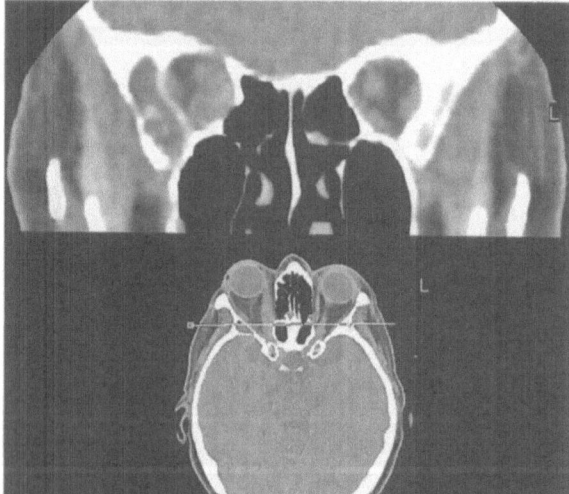

98.7

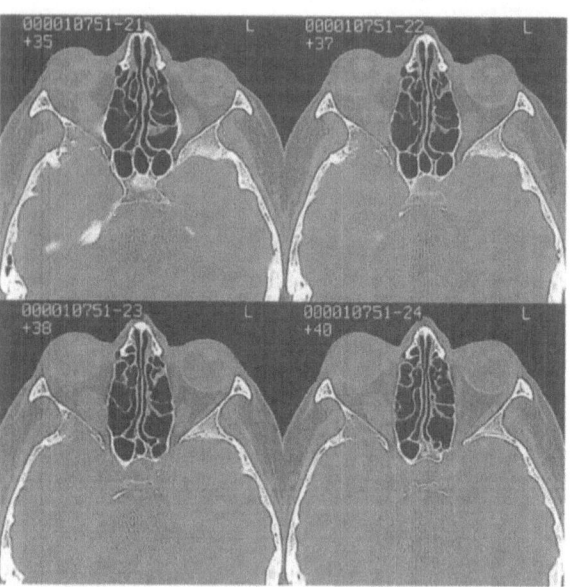

98.8

B. H., 58-year-old man

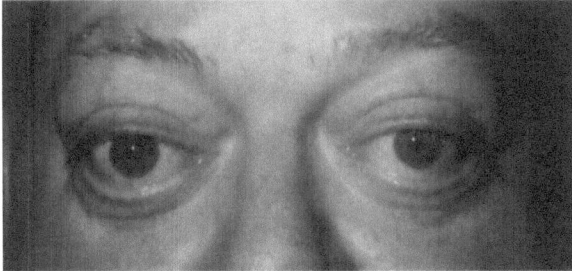

99.1

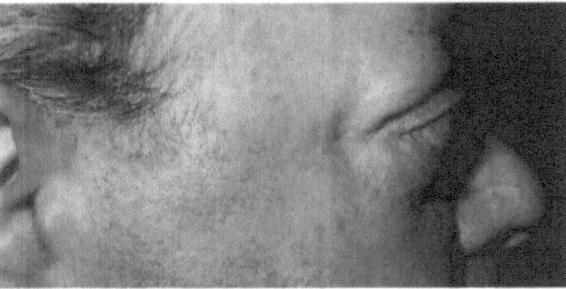

99.2

History and Clinical Findings
Thyroid surgery 20 years ago, since then bilateral protrusion of the globe. Telecobalt therapy of the orbits and repeated radioiodine therapy.

At present, recurrent luxation of the globe. Moderate restriction of ocular motility. Surgical decompression scheduled.

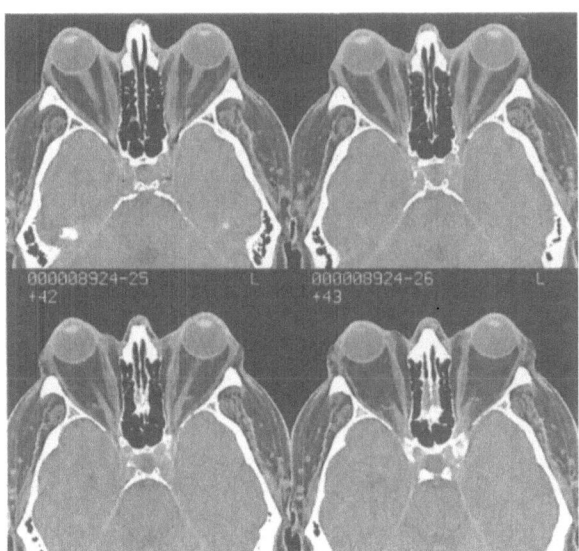

99.3

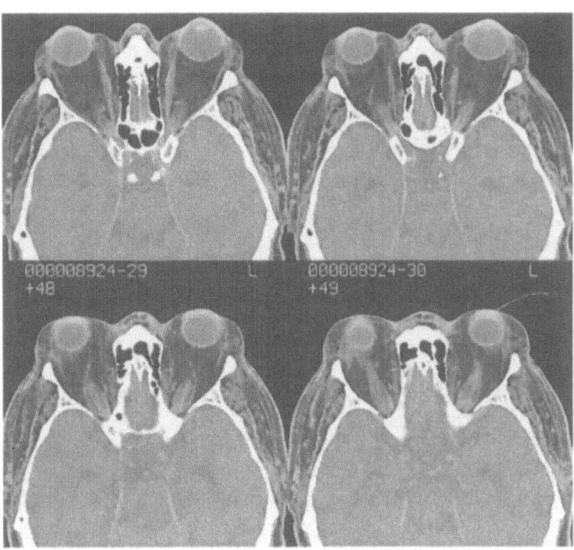

99.4

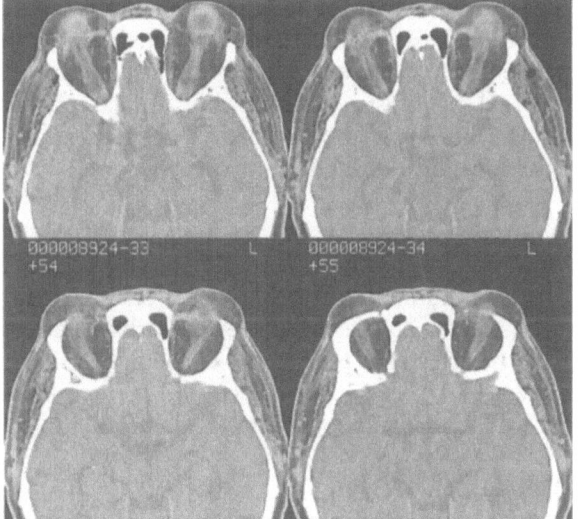

99.5

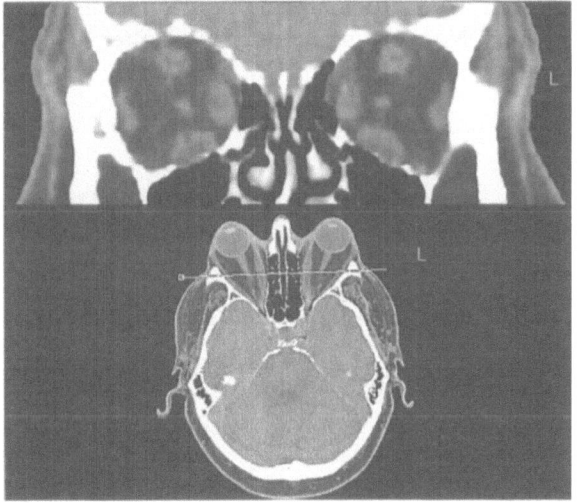

99.6

(Continued on p. 142)

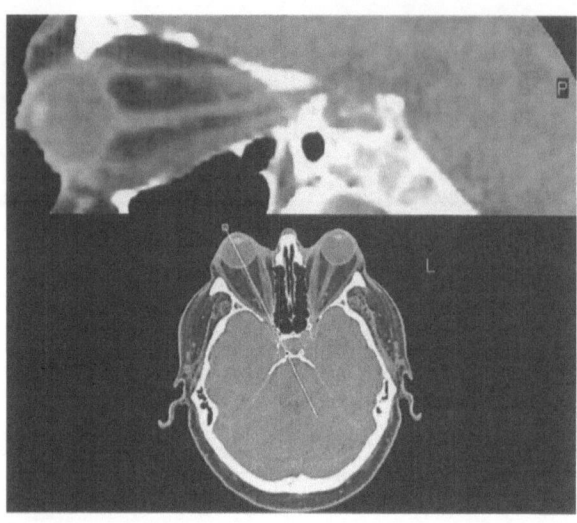

99.7

CT
Slight enlargement of most extraocular muscles. Extended areas of lower density. Considerable increase in the volume of the orbital fat and extreme bilateral proptosis. Considerable increase in the volume of the extraconal orbital fat beneath the right orbital roof. Small bony orbits.

Diagnosis
Polymyositic form of Graves' disease. Fibrotic transformation of extraocular muscles. Considerable increase in the volume of the orbital fat and extreme bilateral proptosis. Particularly in the right orbit, considerable increase in the volume of the extraconal fat beneath the orbital roof.

Clinical Course
Lateral surgical decompression of both orbits. Remission of proptosis and restriction in ocular motility. No more luxations of the globe.

P.H., 56-year-old woman

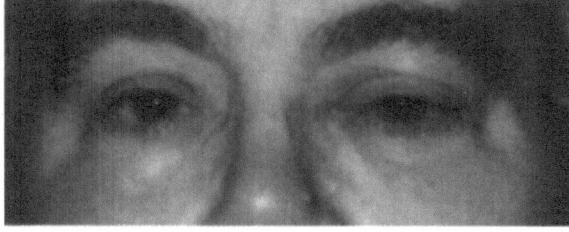

100.1

History and Clinical Findings
Pain in movement of the left eye for 10 days. The optic disc is swollen and hyperemic. Restricted eye movements in left gaze.

CT (100.2, 100.3)
Areas of increased density in the left intraconal space.

Differential Diagnosis
Inflammatory orbital pseudotumor. Metastases of the known carcinoma of the breast (bilateral mastectomy and chemotherapy).

Clinical Course
The patient reported improvement after 1 month of steroid treatment. Four months later, increase in proptosis, no pain.

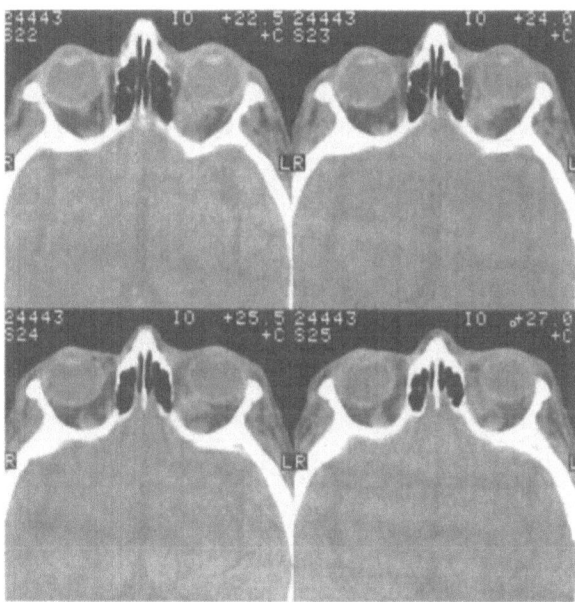

00.2

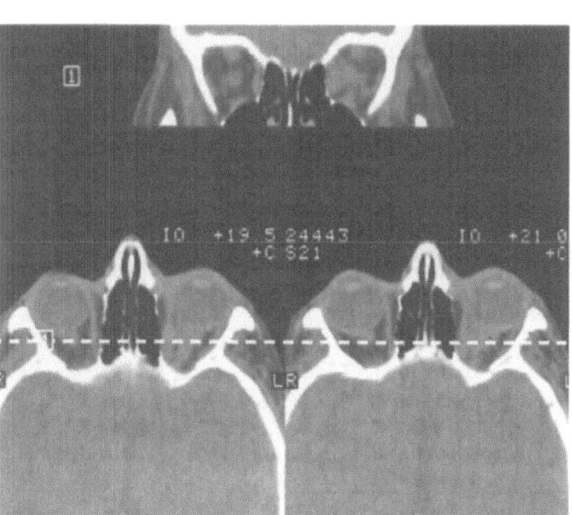

0.3

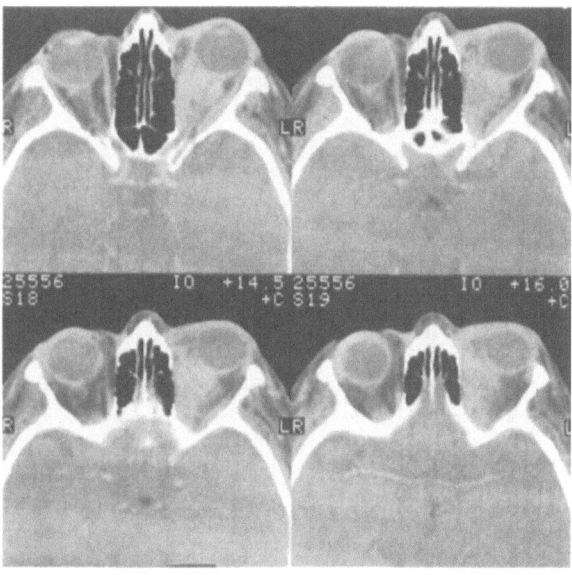

100.4

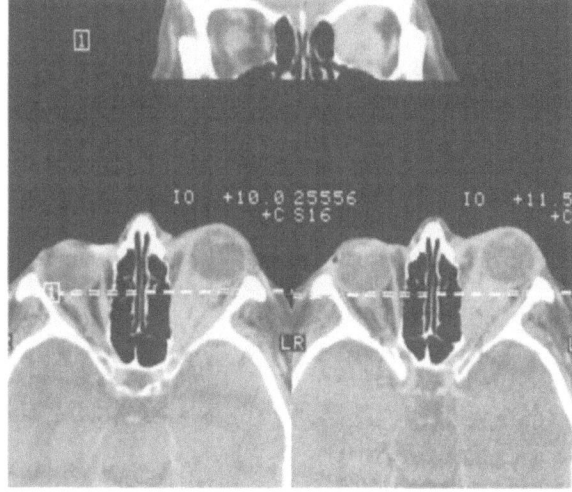

100.5

(Continued on p. 144)

CT (100.4, 100.5):
Extended areas of increased density in the intra-
conal space. Considerable protrusion of the globe.
Orbital structures are masked.

Intracerebral metastases (not shown).

Diagnosis
Metastases of the known carcinoma into the left
orbit.

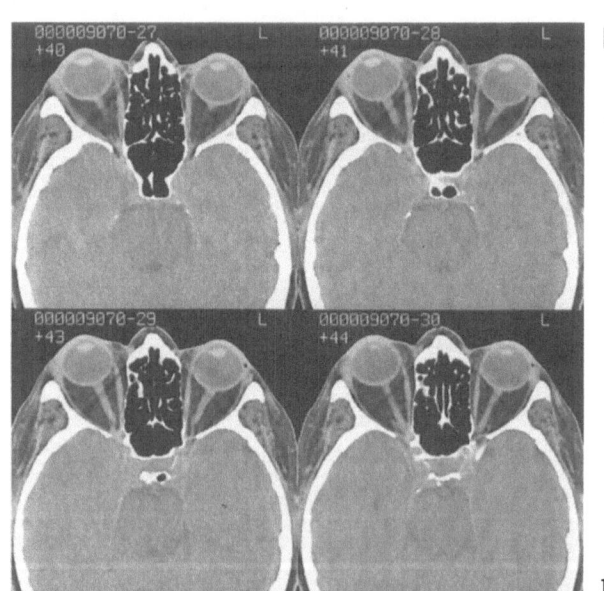

101.1

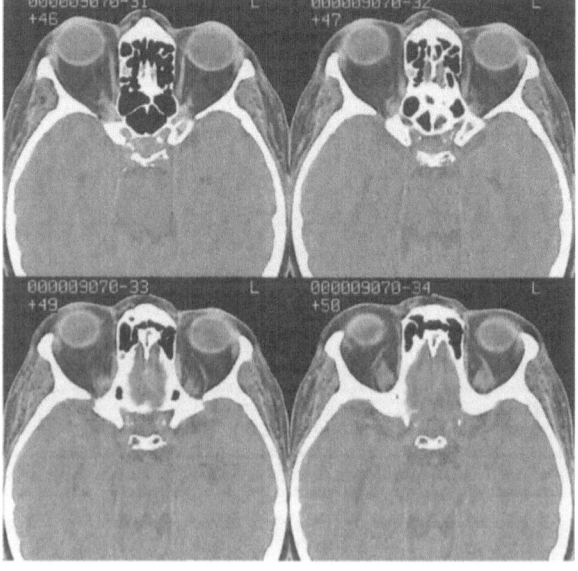

101.2

H. E., 61-year-old woman

History and Clinical Findings

Two years ago, surgery for an aneurysm of the abdominal aorta.

Histopathology: Florid inflammatory and fibrous tissue-producing lesion in the para-aortic connective tissue, with signs of vasculitis. The lesion extends into a para-aortic lymph node, the follicles of which are enlarged. No signs of malignancy.

Three months after surgery, progressive loss of vision in the right eye. Improvement with steroid treatment over a period of 1 year. After discontinuation, progressive visual loss recurred.

Presently, proptosis of the right eye. Visual acuity is reduced to hand movements.

Laboratory signs of inflammation (erythrocyte sedimentation rate, C-reactive protein, circulating immune complexes, and rheumatoid factor) were elevated.

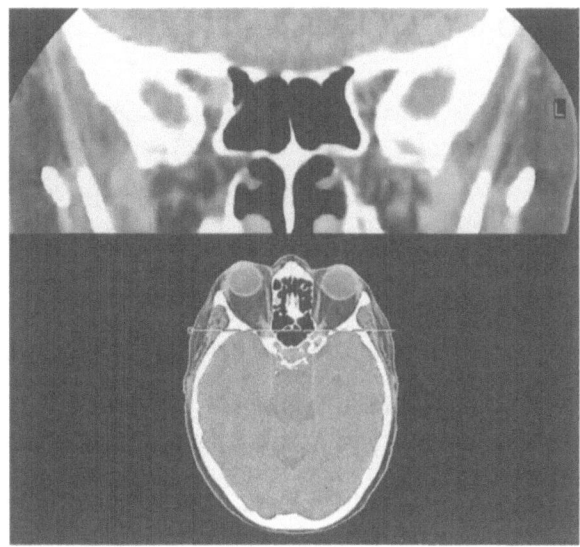

101.5

CT

Small space-occupying lesion in the right orbital apex. Protrusion of the globe.

Diagnosis

In view of the history and the histopathological diagnosis, an inflammatory, vasculitic, fibrotic lesion is the most likely diagnosis.

Comment

If the history had not been known, CT findings might also have been suggestive of a metastasis, or a small tumor in the orbital apex, such as a meningioma.

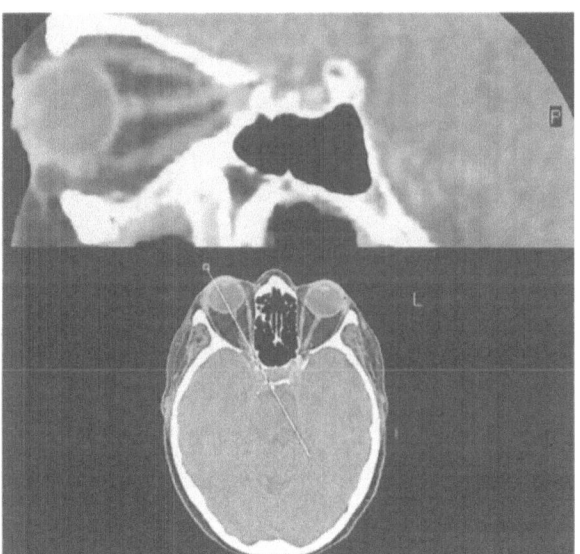

01.3

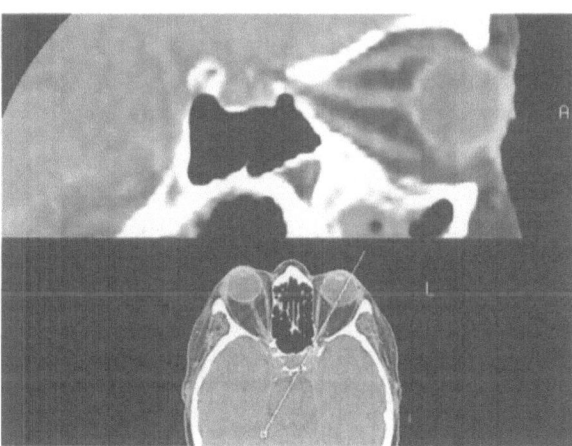

)1.4

V. S., 83-year-old woman

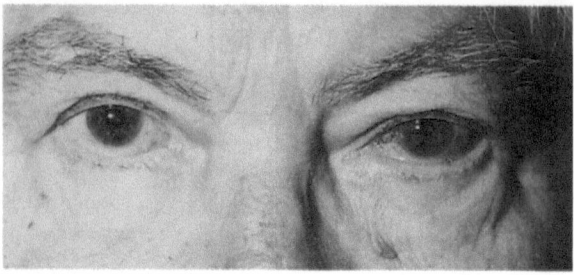

02.1

History and Clinical Findings

"Red eye", episcleral venous injection, elevated intraocular pressure, protrusion of the globe, and periorbital swelling. Diplopia, due to partial oculomotor nerve palsy. Severe headaches.

No improvement of venous congestion after treatment with antibiotic and steroid eye drops. Treatment for elevated intraocular pressure was also ineffective.

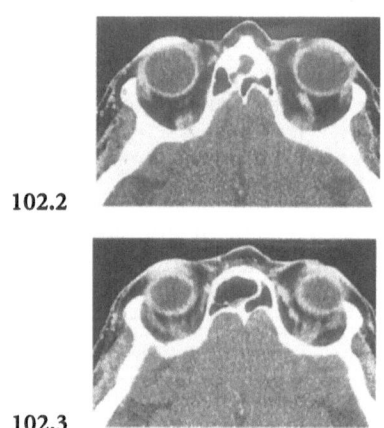

102.2

102.3

CT

Considerable enlargement of the left superior ophthalmic vein and of the left supratrochlear vein.

Diagnosis

Findings are highly suspicious of a cavernous sinus fistula.

Duplex Sonography

Typical flow reversal in the supratrochlear vein.

Angiography

Arterio-venous dural fistula within the cavernous sinus.

Clinical Course

Complete remission of signs and symptoms after transvenous occlusion of the fistula via the petrosal sinus (Courtesy Professor D. Kühne, Chief of Department of Radiology and Neuroradiology, Alfried Krupp Hospital, Essen, Germany).

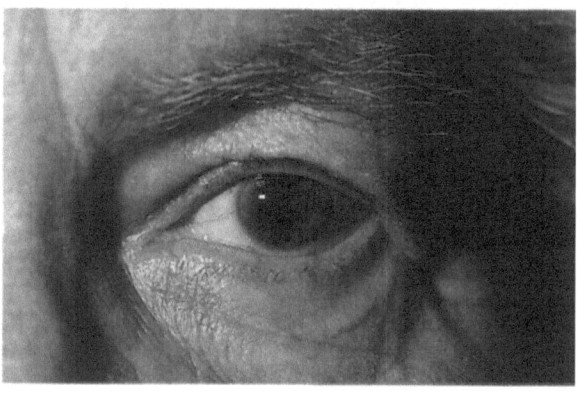

102.4

Postoperatively, complete remission of clinical signs and symptoms (102.4).

H. E., 38-year-old man

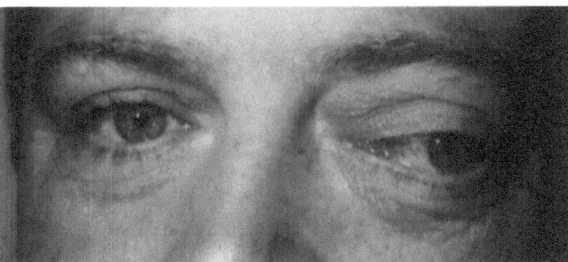

03.1

History and Clinical Findings
Orbital pain, protrusion of the left globe and diplopia for 7 weeks. Steroid treatment.

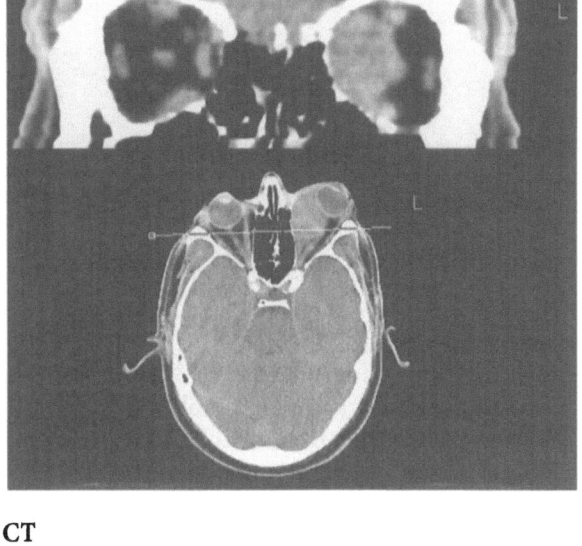

103.4

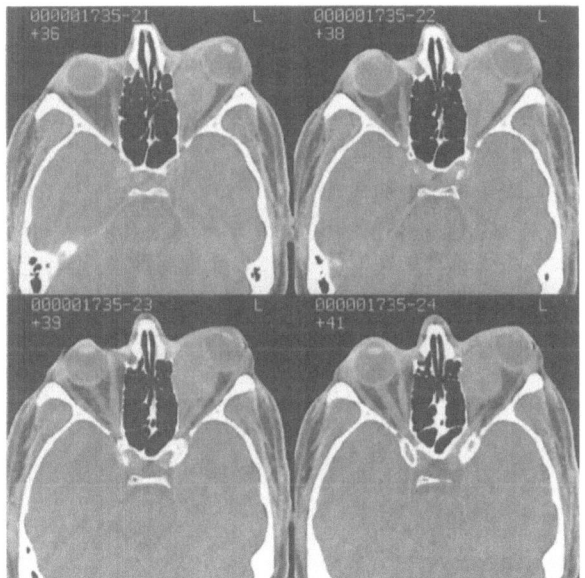

03.2

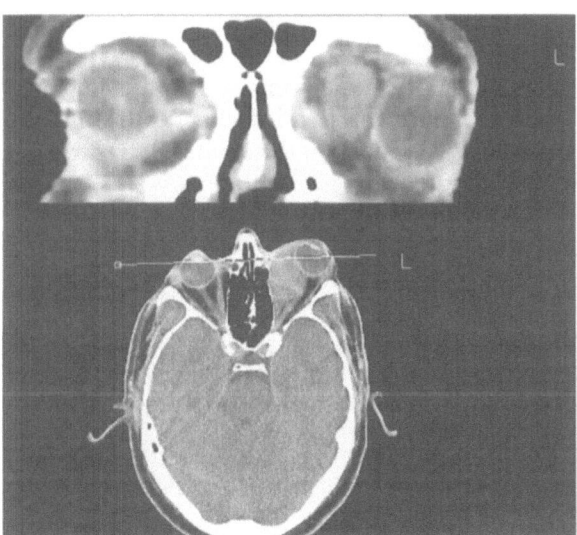

3.3

CT
Large, spindle-shaped, space-occupying lesion in the left medial rectus muscle. The adjacent bone is excavated but not destroyed. The adjacent part of the wall of the globe is flattened. Considerable protrusion of the left globe.

Differential Diagnosis
Myositic form of inflammatory orbital pseudotumor or malignant neoplasm. A surgical biopsy is necessary.

Histopathology
Rhabdomyosarcoma.

G. H., 72-year-old woman

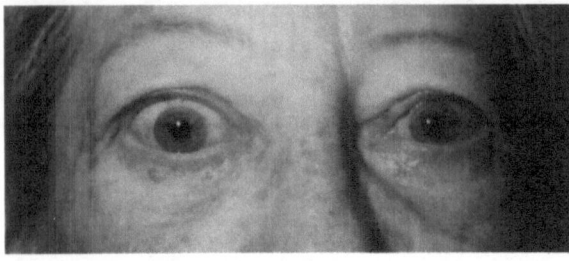

104.1

History and Clinical Findings

Hyperthyroid episodes 9, 10, and 12 years ago, associated with deaths in the family.

Antithyroid medication for the past 12 months.

Proptosis of the right eye, lid retraction and diplopia for 5 weeks.

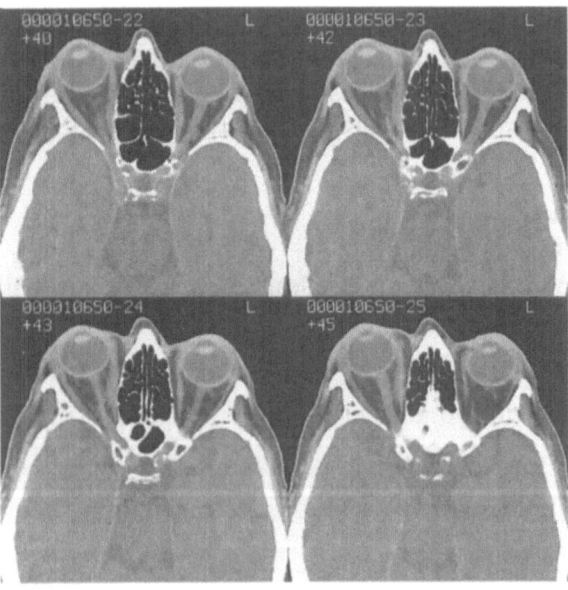

104.2

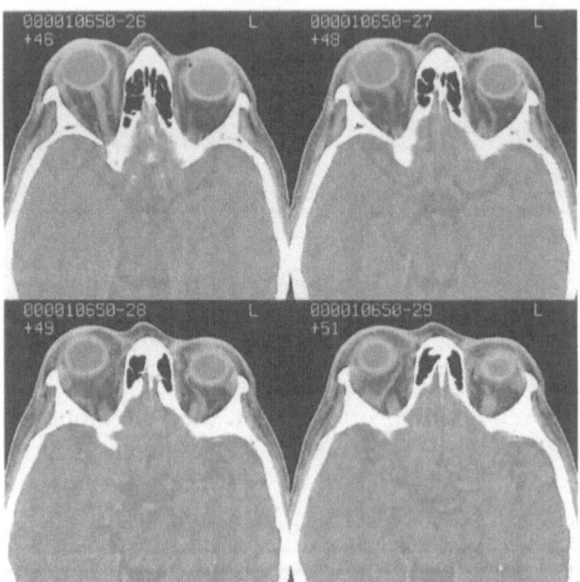

104.3

104.4

CT

Unilateral enlargement of most extraocular muscles, particularly of the inferior rectus muscle. Increase in the volume of the orbital fat. Protrusion of the right globe.

Diagnosis

Unilateral polymyositic form of Graves' disease.

Clinical Course

Remission of symptoms after irradiation of the orbital apex.

D. J., 57-year-old man

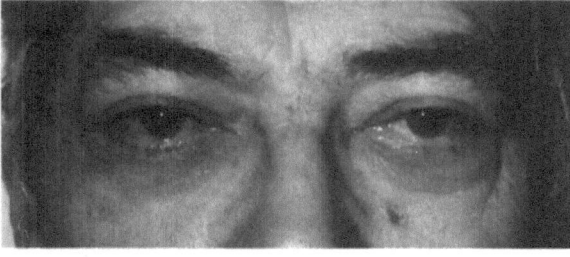

05.1

History and Clinical Findings

The patient was previously diagnosed with non-Hodgkin lymphoma.

Increasing proptosis, more prominent on the right side, chemosis and, occasionally, diplopia for the past 4 weeks. Corrected vision 100/100.

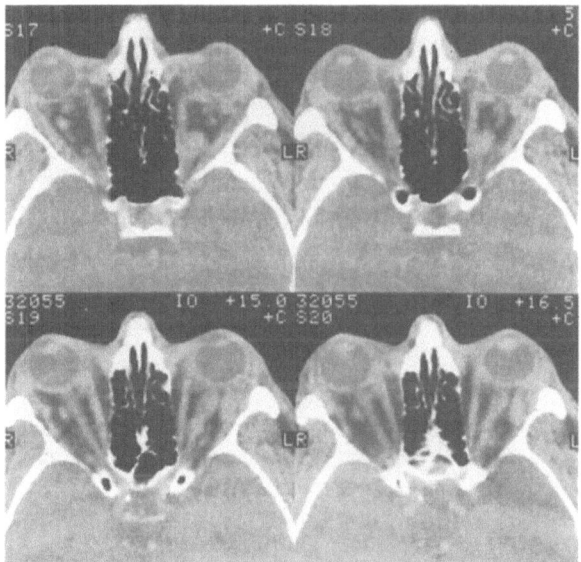

05.2

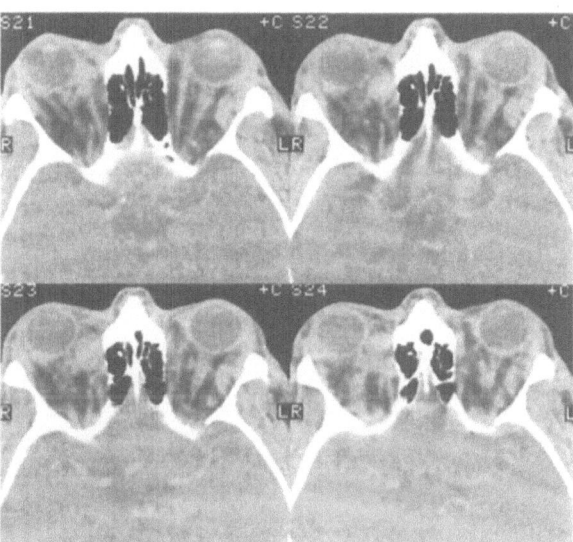

05.3

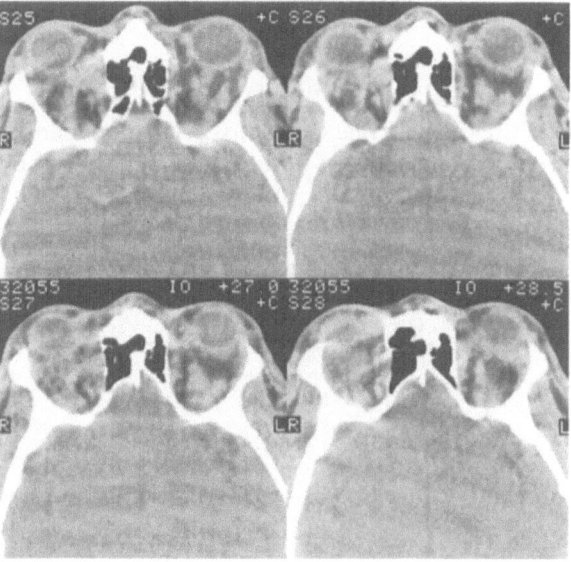

105.4

CT

Multiple, irregular areas of increased density within the retrobulbar spaces. Moderate enlargement of extraocular muscles. Bilateral proptosis.

Diagnosis

With the history of non-Hodgkin lymphoma, most probably bilateral metastatic infiltration.

Histopathology

Centrocytic-centroblastic non-Hodgkin lymphoma.

Clinical Course

Telecobalt radiation of both retrobulbar spaces (20 Gy) was followed by marked improvement.

M. G., 39-year-old woman

History and Clinical Findings
For the past 2 years, proptosis and, on bending over, brief episodes of blurred vision in the left eye.

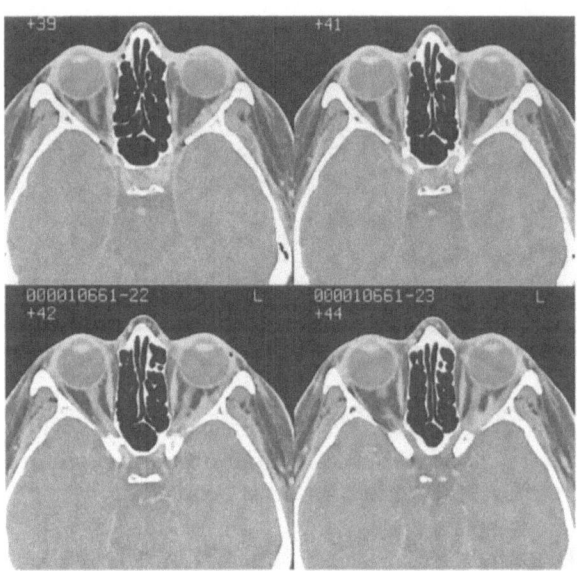

106.1

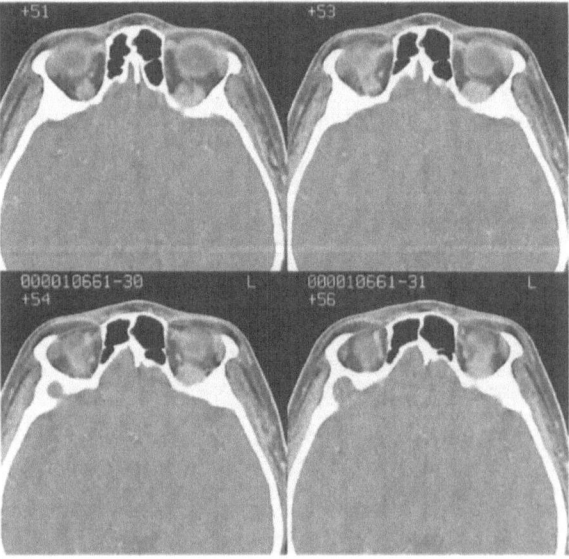

106.2

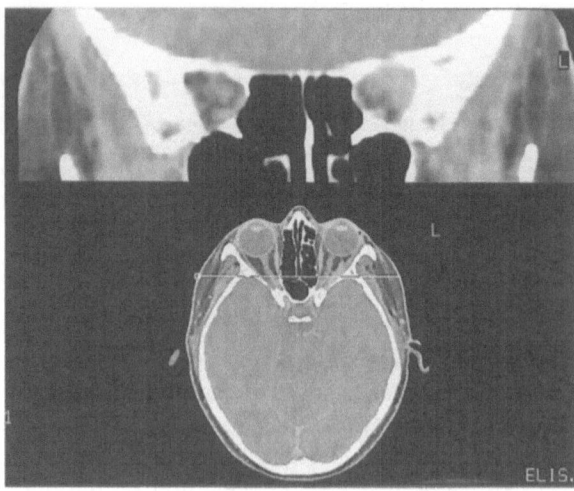

106.3

CT (106.1 – 106.3)
Scans with the patient lying on her back.
   Small, flat area of increased density within the left superior and lateral extraconal space.

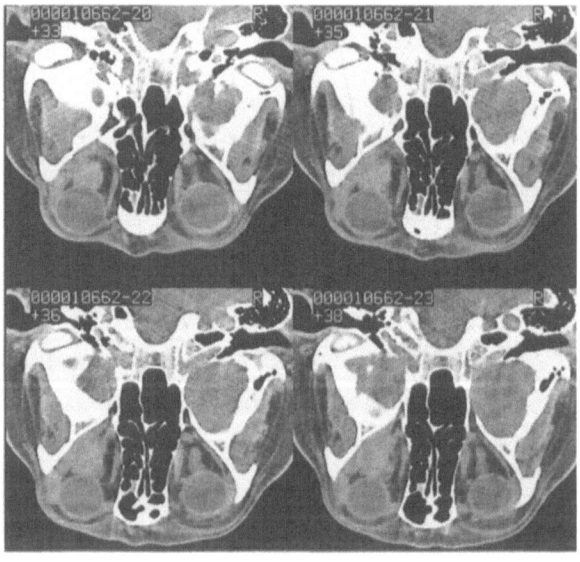

106.4

(Continued on p. 151)

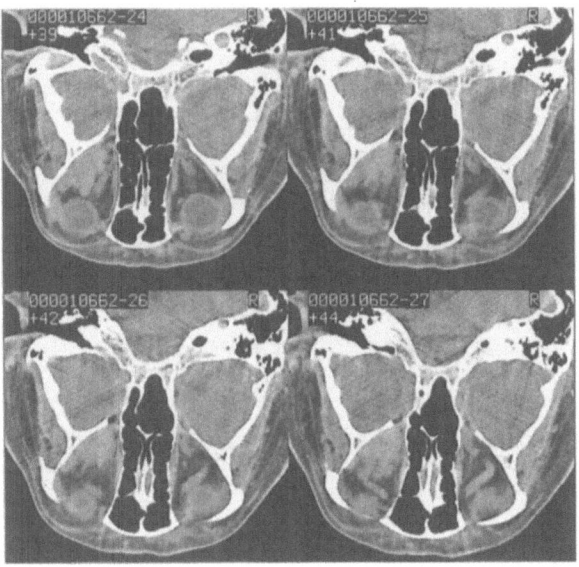

06.5

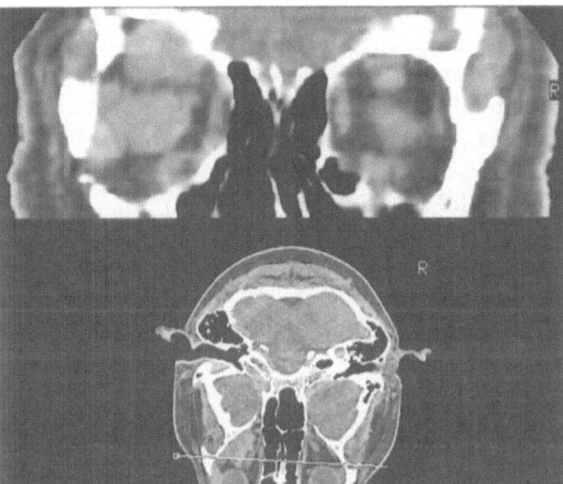

06.6

CT (106.5, 106.6)
Scans with the patient's head positioned downward.

Large, polycyclic, hyperdense, space-occupying lesion and considerable excavation of the adjacent orbital roof. Compared to the scans obtained in conventional technique, considerably greater size of the soft-tissue lesion.

Diagnosis
Venous malformation in the left orbit.

Comment
With no knowledge of the clinical symptoms, the CT findings could also have been interpreted as a form of inflammatory orbital pseudotumor or as another soft-tissue lesion. On CT scans obtained with the patient's head positioned downward, diagnosis of venous malformation could clearly be established.

H. D., 38-year-old woman

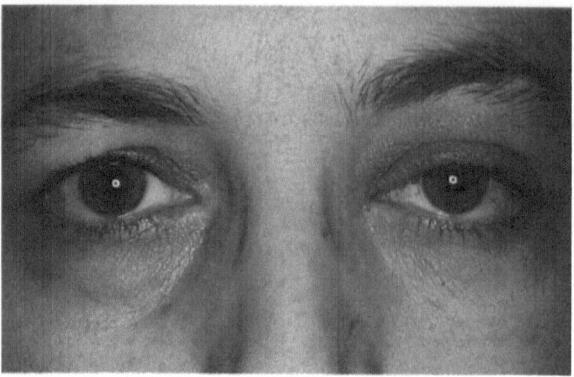

107.1

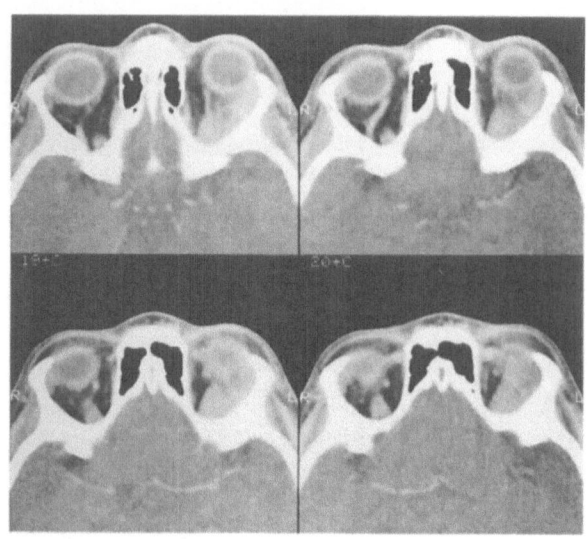

107.3

History and Clinical Findings
For the past 4 months, swelling of the left lids, initially painless, later intermittent pain. At present, slight swelling and hyperemia of the left upper lid, ptosis, and protrusion of the globe.

CT
Homogeneous soft-tissue lesion in the left superior and lateral extraconal space. The tumor cannot be delineated clearly against the lacrimal gland, the lateral rectus muscle, and the upper muscle complex.

Differential Diagnosis
Chronic inflammation or lymphatic disease.

Histopathology
Fibrous tissue-producing inflammation with focal fibrinoid necroses.

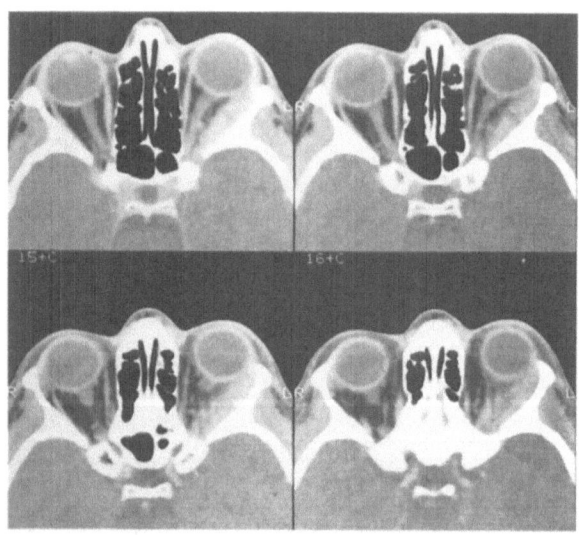

107.2

R. J., 49-year-old man

History and Clinical Findings
Lid swelling, proptosis and restricted motility of the right eye for 6 years. Partial remission of proptosis and of the limitation of upward gaze with steroid treatment. After each dose reduction, however, symptoms recurred.

CT 4 years ago: Considerable enlargement of the extraocular muscles of the right eye and of the right lacrimal gland.

Three months ago, for the first time, papilledema and congestion of the retinal veins in the right eye and decrease in visual acuity (from 100/100 to 60/100).

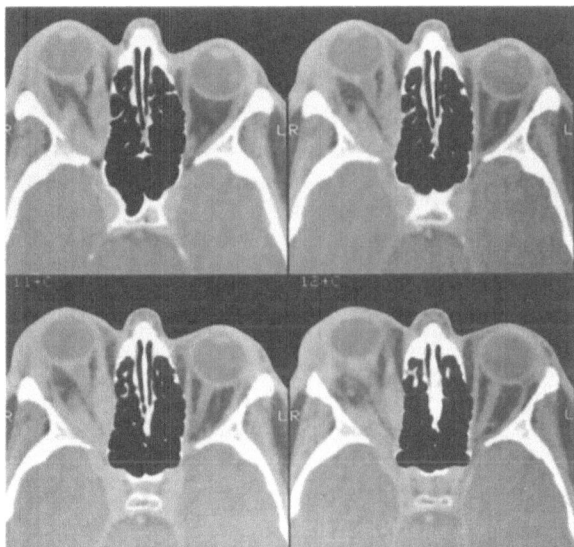

08.1

08.2

CT (108.1, 108.2)
Considerable enlargement of most extraocular muscles in the right orbit. The optic nerve appears to be compressed in the orbital apex. Considerable enlargement of the walls of the right globe. Extended, striated areas of increased density within the orbital fat. Enlargement of the optic nerve sheath. Considerable enlargement of the lacrimal gland and of the periorbital tissues. The areas of increased density extend into the cavernous sinus via the orbital fissure.

Differential Diagnosis
Inflammatory orbital pseudotumor or systemic lymphatic disease.

Clinical Course
Surgical biopsy: Benign lymphatic hyperplasia, consistent with the diagnosis of inflammatory orbital pseudotumor.

Radiation therapy (20 Gy) was followed by partial remission of ptosis, as well as by a reduction of ocular hypertension.

Four months later, remission of proptosis and diplopia.

Ocular motility normal.

(Continued on p. 154)

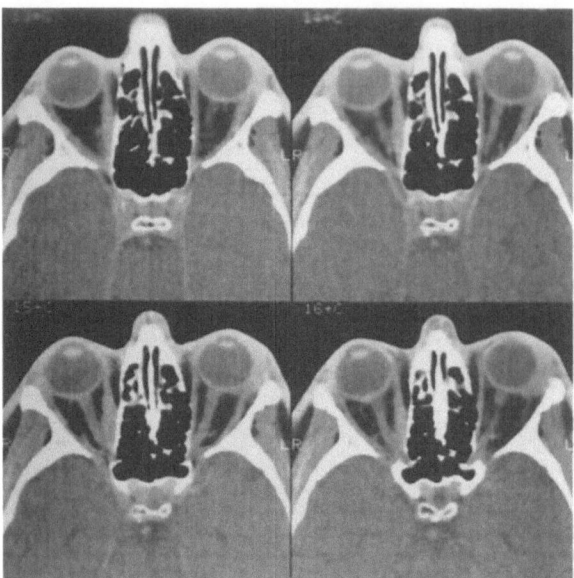

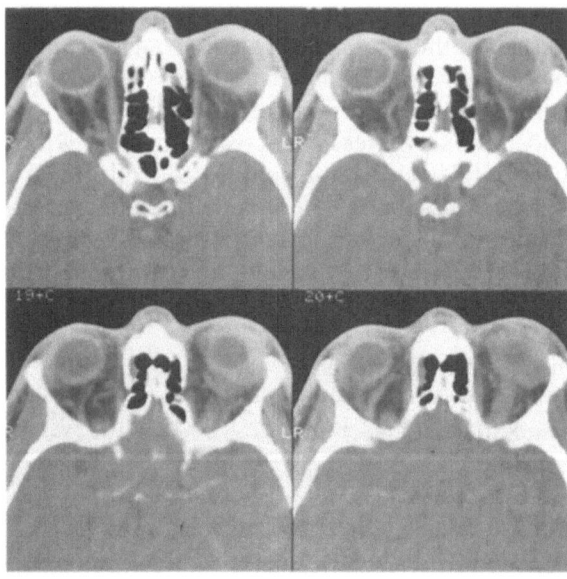

08.3

08.4

CT (108.3, 108.4)
Fifteen months later: Slight enlargement of the
right extraocular muscles. The right lacrimal gland
is poorly defined, the left lacrimal gland is considerably enlarged. Considerable enlargement of
the wall of the globe. Slight enlargement of periorbital soft tissue.

Diagnosis
Inflammatory orbital pseudotumor, histopatholo-
gically benign lymphatic hyperplasia.
    Considerable improvement in the right eye.
Deterioration in the left eye.

S. A., 51-year-old woman

History and Clinical Findings
Progressive proptosis and painful swelling of the left temporal upper lid for the past 3 years. Lateral orbitotomy and partial removal of the tumor performed elsewhere.

Increasing protrusion of the left globe for the past 4 months.

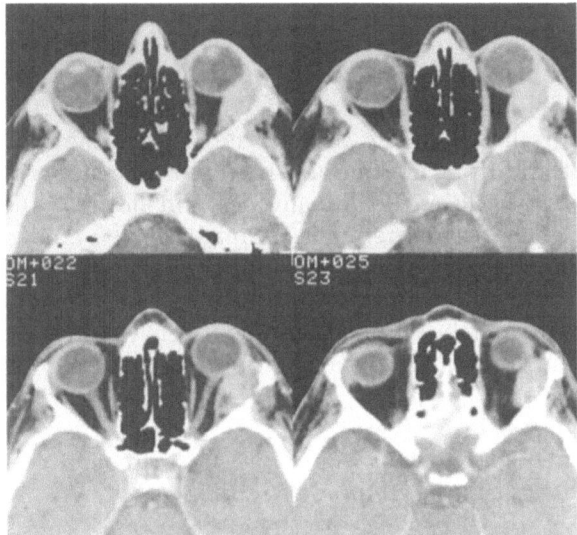

09.1

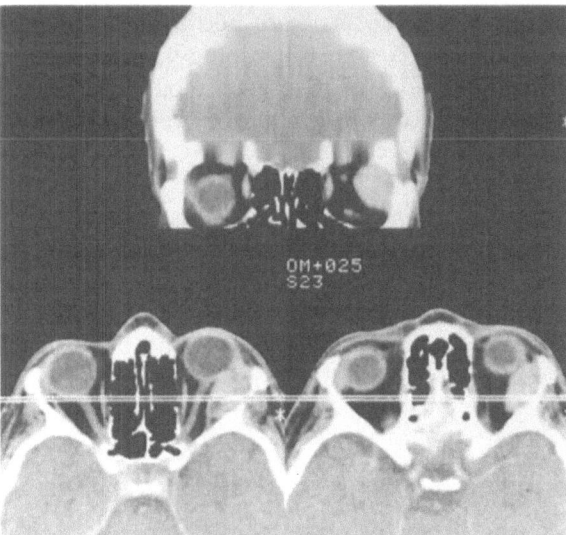

09.2

CT
Large, roundish, inhomogeneous, space-occupying lesion in the left lacrimal fossa, pressing on the globe. Within the lesion, roundish, hypodense areas. Medial displacement of the globe and the lateral rectus muscle.

Diagnosis
Growth of the residual tumor.

Clinical Course
Exenteration of the orbit including the adjacent bone.

Histopathology: Adenoid cystic carcinoma of the lacrimal gland.

Recurrence of the tumor 1 year later.

Partial resection of the maxilla followed by radiation therapy.

Comment
The initial operation should have been performed as a one-stage en-bloc-resection.

B. J., 78-year-old man

History and Clinical Findings
Vision in the right eye was reduced to light percep-
tion, vision in the left eye was 80/100. Right optic
disc swelling.

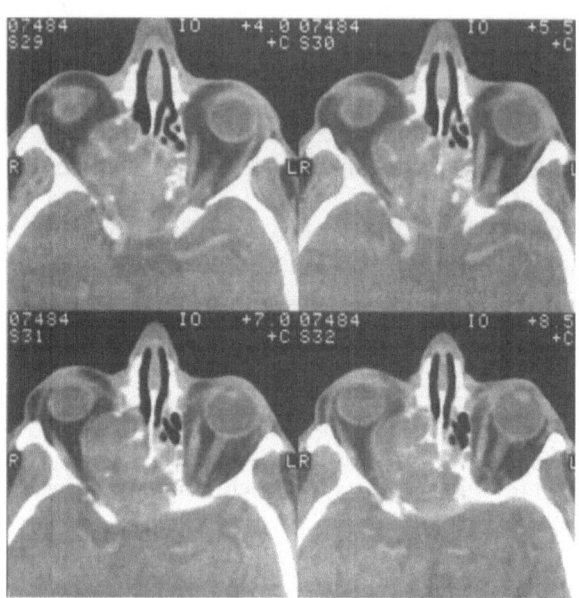

10.1

CT
Large, solid lesion, occupying both ethmoidal
air cells and both sphenoid sinuses. The tumor
invades the right nasal cavity and, to a lesser
extent, the right maxillary sinus. The right medial
orbital wall is destroyed, the tumor invades the
orbit displacing the medial rectus muscle. The
dorsal part of the muscle cannot be delineated
clearly from the tumor. The tumor displaces the
right optic nerve and invades and destroys the
right optic foramen. The left medial wall is eroded
but not completely destroyed. The left optic canal
is slightly invaded by the tumor. The sphenoid
plane and the sellar floor are completely destroyed.
The tumor invades the anterior cranial fossa.

Diagnosis
Solid space-occupying lesion, most probably originating in the ethmoidal air cells.

Clinical Course
Two surgical biopsies were performed 6 months
ago, 4 weeks apart. Histopathology: Mucoceles.
   Histopathology of a surgical biopsy performed
after the CT scans shown above: Well-differentiat-
ed mucinous carcinoma.

Comment
The histopathological diagnosis of a mucocele
must be followed by diagnostic imaging, since
primary malignant lesions can frequently lead to
secondary mucoceles by obstructing the ostia of
the sinuses affected.

J. C., 28-year-old woman

History and Clinical Findings

Six months ago, the pregnant patient was diagnosed with enlargement of both lacrimal glands, initially more pronounced on the left side.

Delivery 4 months ago, subsequent steroid treatment. Recurrence of the enlargement after discontinuation of steroid treatment.

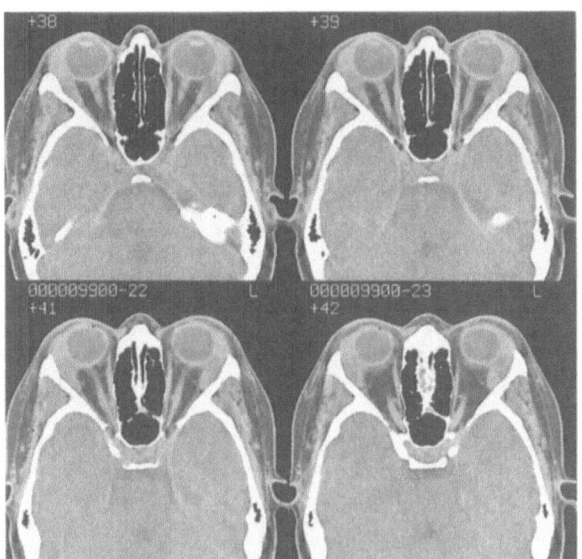

11.1

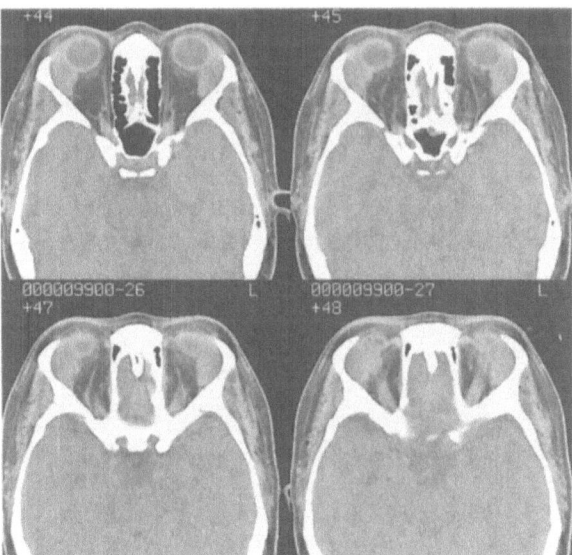

11.2

CT
Symmetrical enlargement of both lacrimal glands, extending anteriorly and dorsally deeply into the lateral extraconal space. Bilateral protrusion of the globe.

Differential Diagnosis
Leukemic infiltration or dacryoadenitic form of inflammatory orbital pseudotumor.

Histopathology
Granulomatous dacryoadenitis.

Comment
The form of the enlargement, a homogeneous swelling with the original form being retained, makes the diagnosis of a mixed tumor or a carcinoma of the lacrimal gland highly unlikely.

Systemic inflammatory disease, tuberculosis, sarcoidosis, and lymphoproliferative disease were excluded.

F. C., 39-year-old woman

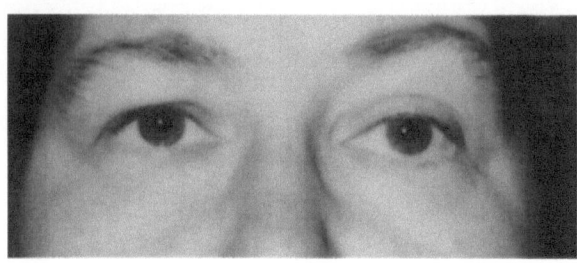

112.1

History and Clinical Findings

Recurrent "optic neuritis" in the left eye over a period of 1 year. Good response to steroid treatment, with recurrences, however, after each dose reduction.

Presently, pain and protrusion of the globe. Optic nerve atrophy, vision was reduced to 10/100. Afferent pupillary defect.

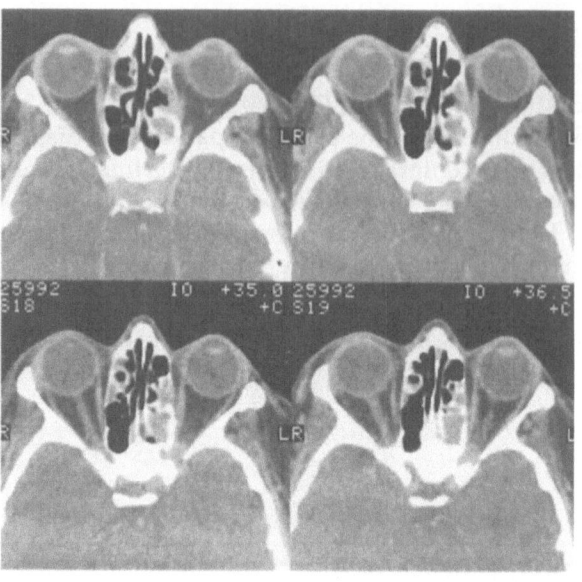

112.2

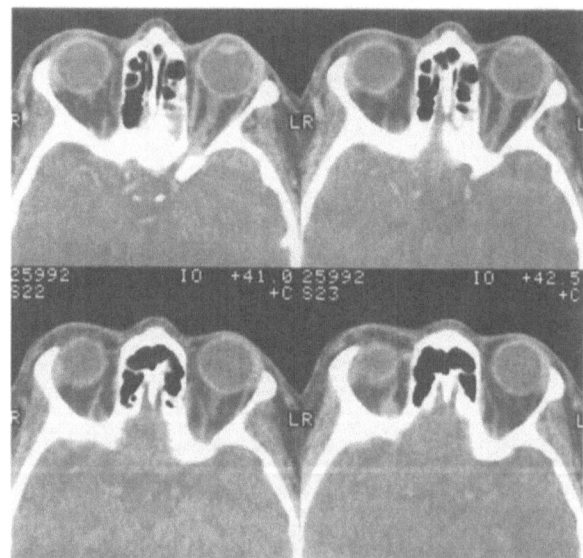

112.3

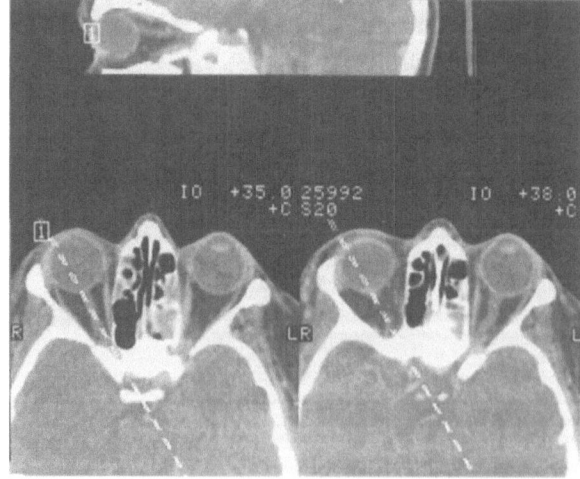

(Continued on p. 159)

112.4

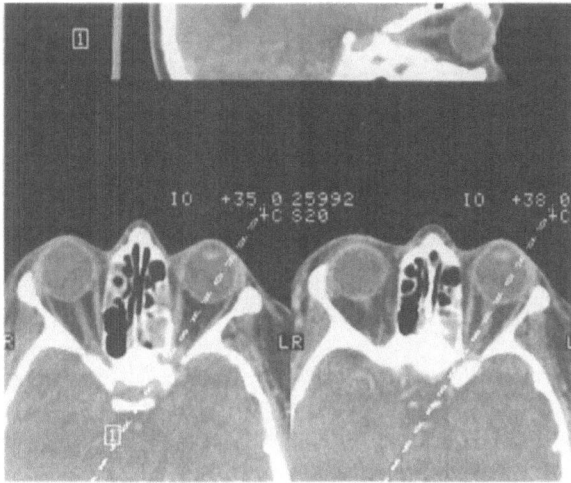

12.5

CT

State after surgery on the ethmoidal air cells and the maxillary sinus. Hyperostoses in these areas with soft-tissue margins.

Soft tissue within the left posterior ethmoidal air cells and within the left sphenoid sinus. Bone defect in the superior and anterior part of the wall of the sphenoid sinus, from where the soft-tissue mass extends into the orbital apex.

Diagnosis

Small space-occupying lesion in the left posterior ethmoidal air cells and in the left sphenoid sinus, extending into the orbital apex.

Endonasal biopsy: Inflammatory tissue with perivascular infiltration suggestive of vasculitis.

Laboratory tests confirmed Wegener's granulomatosis.

Clinical Course

Remission of symptoms with immunosuppressive therapy with cyclophosphamide and steroids.

Two years after its initiation, the patient discontinued the immunosuppressive medication. Subsequently, she developed further symptoms of Wegener's granulomatosis including rapid progressive glomerulonephritis. Increase in the concentration of autoantibodies (c-ANCA) and recurrence of the "optic neuritis".

Comment

The patient's history and the bone defects indicate that the lesion originates in a paranasal sinus. A meningioma of the orbital apex can thus be excluded.

G. E., 36-year-old woman

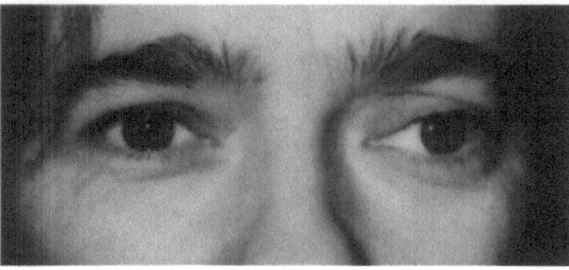

113.1

History and Clinical Findings
The patient was diagnosed with cancer of the breast 1 year ago. Radiation and chemotherapy in Kazakhstan.

Proptosis for the past 3 months.

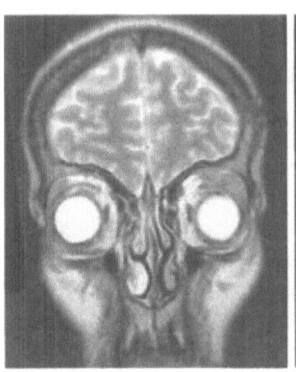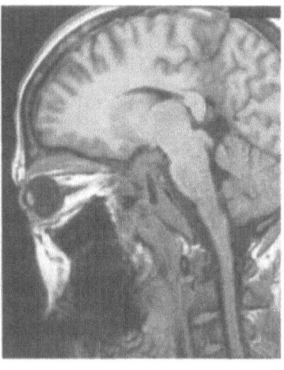

.2 – 3

MRI (113.2, 113.3)
Space-occupying lesion in the superior and lateral extraconal space.

Diagnosis
Metastasis of the known carcinoma of the breast.

Clinical Course
Bilateral mastectomy followed by chemotherapy for multiple bone metastases.

Blurred vision 9 months later. No pain.

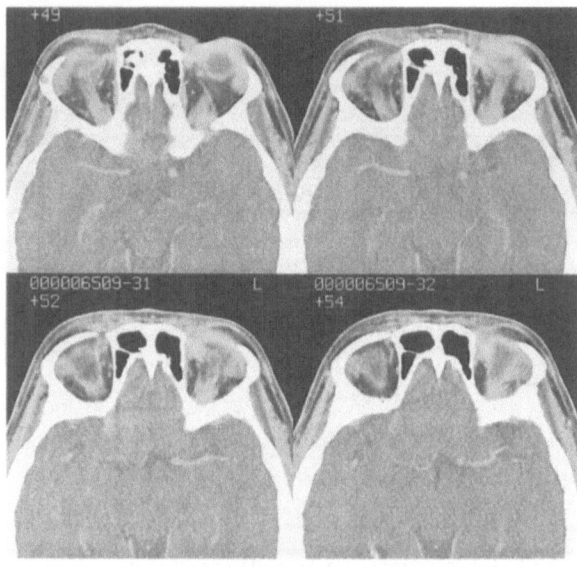

113.4

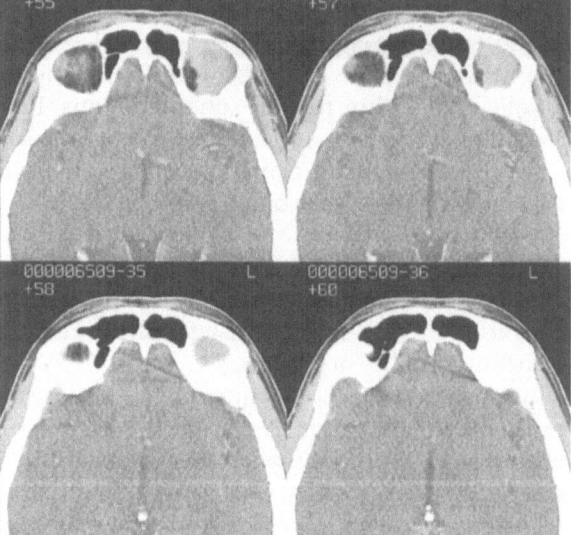

113.5

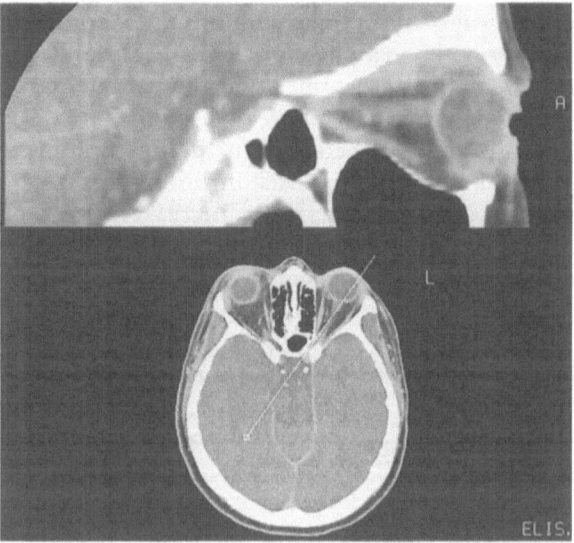

113.6

(Continued on p. 161)

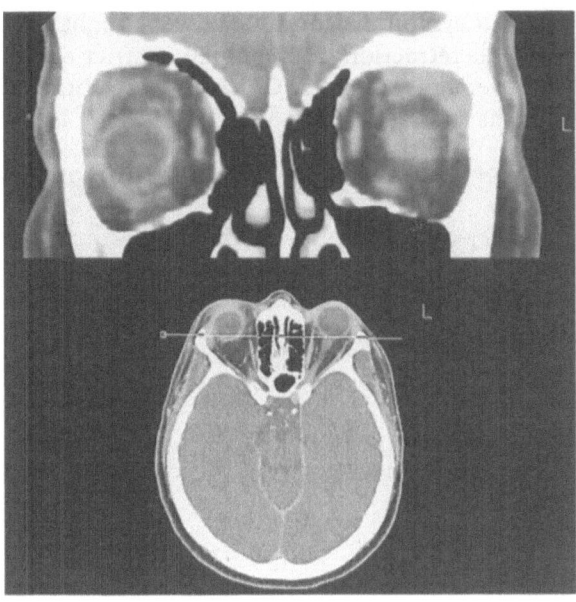

13.7

CT (113.4–113.7)
Soft-tissue mass in the superior and lateral extra-conal space, causing the superior rectus muscle to be displaced caudally. Slight protrusion of the globe.

Diagnosis
No change in the size of the metastasis in the superior and lateral extraconal space.

J. F., 68-year-old man

History and Clinical Findings
Cataract surgery 2 days ago.

Postoperatively vertical diplopia. Limitation of upward and downward gaze in the right eye.

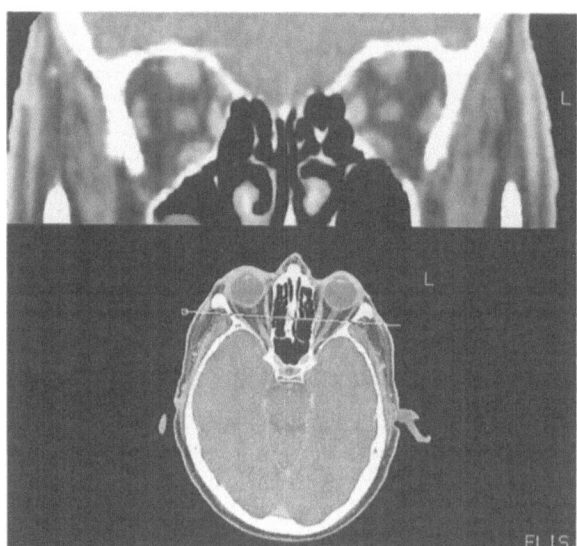

114.1

CT (114.1)
Slight enlargement of the right superior rectus muscle.

Differential Diagnosis
Hematoma within the right superior rectus muscle due to retrobulbar anesthesia, or monomyositic form of Graves' disease, or ocular myositis.

Clinical Course
Diagnostic tests regarding thyroid disease, including assessment of antibodies, were negative. Spontaneous improvement of clinical signs and symptoms.

Due to symptoms in the *left* eye – slight proptosis, lid retraction and complex restrictions of eye movements – further CT scans were obtained 8 months later.

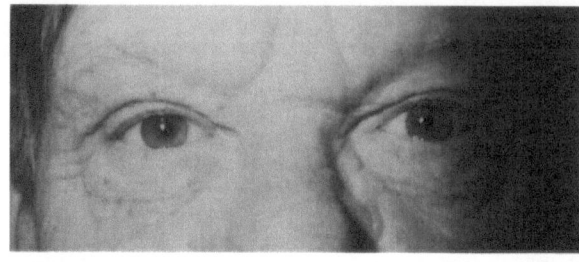

114.2

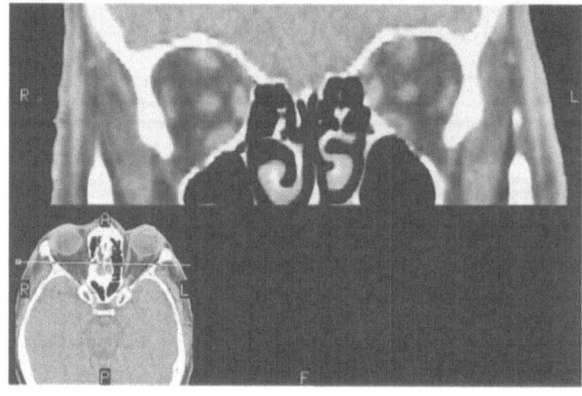

114.3

CT (114.2, 114.3)
Enlargement of the right superior rectus muscle can no longer be visualized.

In contrast to the previous scans, the *left* superior rectus muscle is enlarged.

Diagnosis
The clinical course points to the myositic form of inflammatory orbital pseudotumor.

Comment
Restricted ocular motility is not likely to have been brought about by retrobulbar anesthesia. Due to the poor vision, double vision was probably not perceived before cataract surgery.

S. E., 67-year-old woman

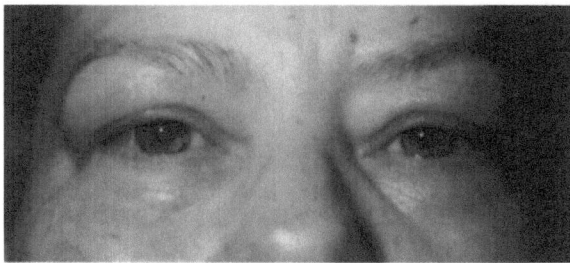

15.1

History and Clinical Findings

Autoimmune thyroiditis was diagnosed 11 years ago. Two courses of radioiodine therapy, 11 years ago and again 2 years ago. Presently the patient is euthyroid. No symptoms according to the patient.

Considerable lid swelling, in particular of the temporal parts of both upper lids.

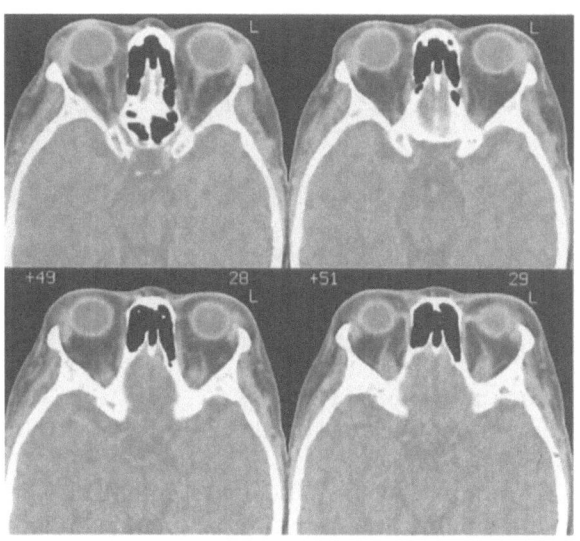

115.3

CT

Moderate increase in the volume of the orbital fat and slight enlargement of most extraocular muscles. Bilateral enlargement and protrusion of the lacrimal gland, particularly of the palpebral portion.

Diagnosis

Predominantly dacryoadenitic form of Graves' disease.

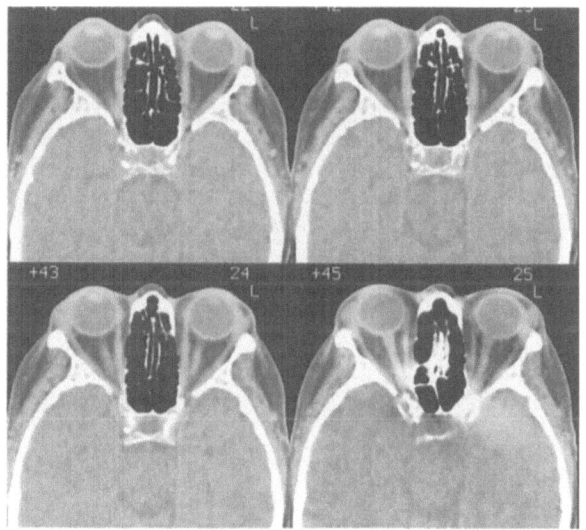

15.2

K. L., 69-year-old woman

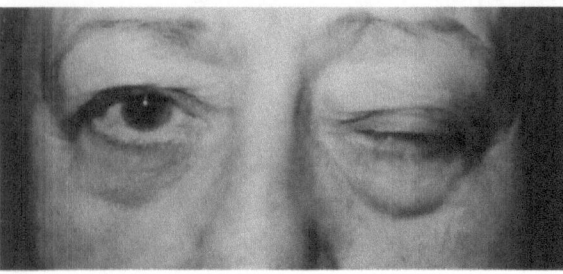

116.1

History and Clinical Findings
Amputation of the left breast 18 months ago. Ptosis and proptosis.

Six months ago, the patient was euthyroid.

One month ago, removal of an enlarged lymph node in the left supraclavicular fossa and initiation of chemotherapy.

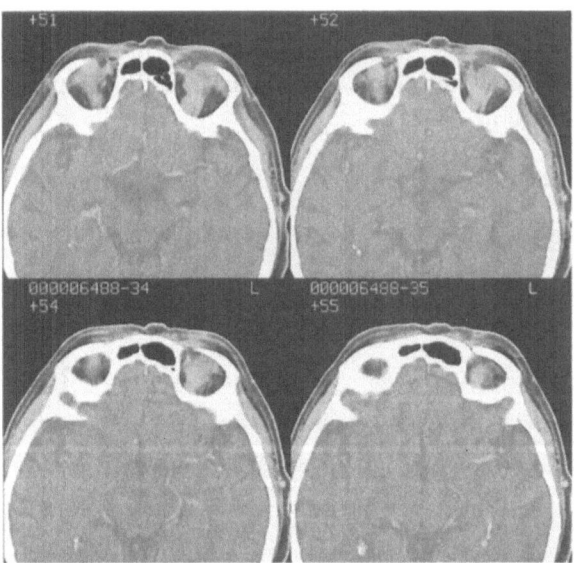

116.2

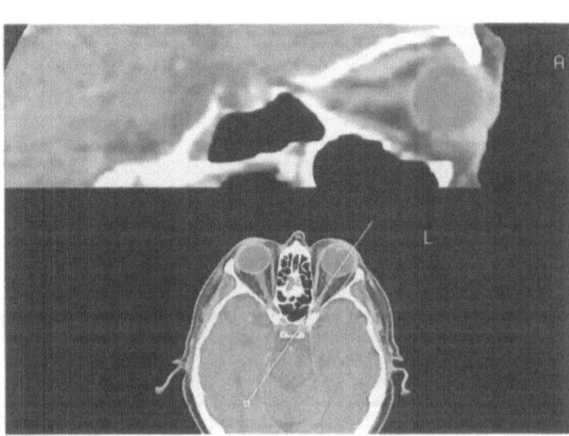

116.3

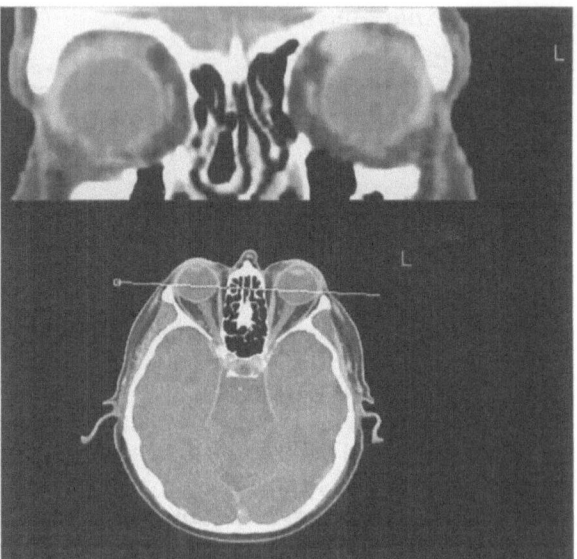

116.4

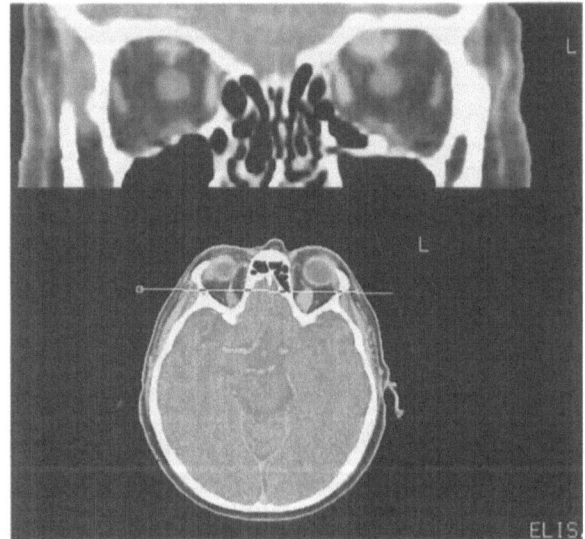

116.5

CT
Enlargement of the left levator palpebrae and superior rectus muscle.

Differential Diagnosis
State after monomyositic form of Graves' disease and myasthenic reaction.

A metastasis does not seem a likely diagnosis due to the relatively homogeneous, spindle-shaped enlargement of the upper muscle complex, and to the long clinical course.

Clinical Course
No change in findings 2 years later.

P.H., 57-year-old female

History and Clinical Findings

The patient complains of swelling around the right eye, hyperlacrimation and a burning sensation for the past 6 months. Protrusion of the right globe, episcleral and retinal venous congestion.

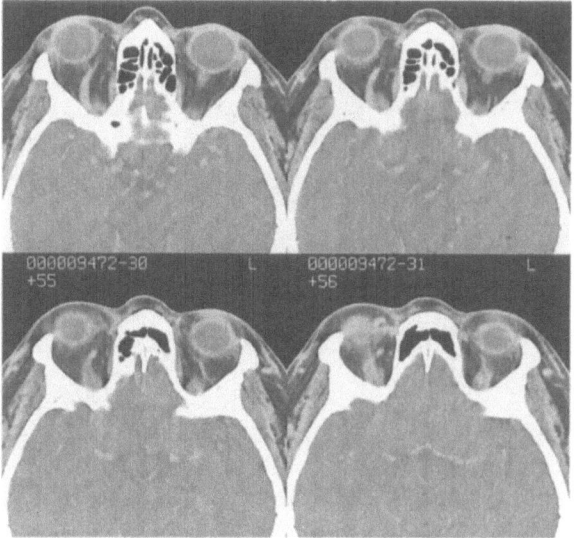

117.2

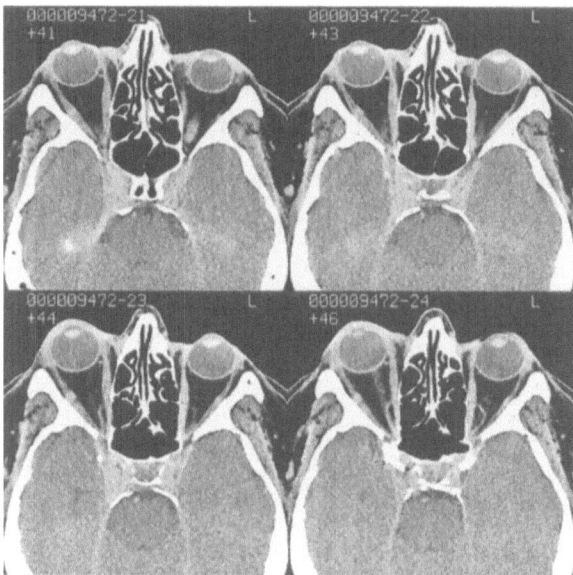

17.1

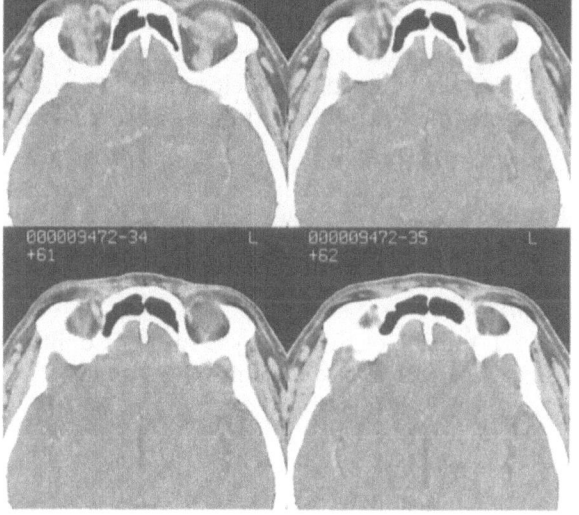

117.3

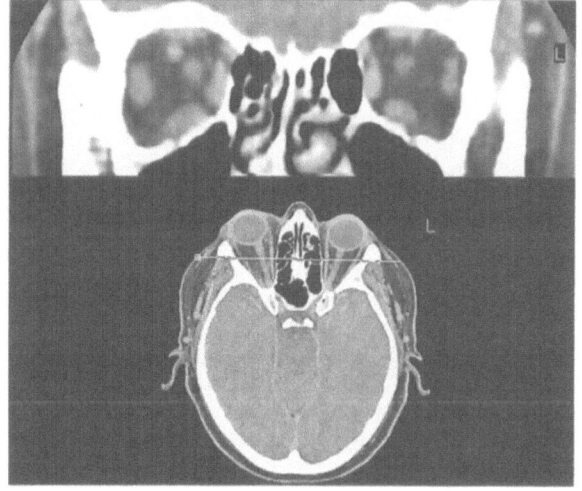

117.4

(Continued on p. 166)

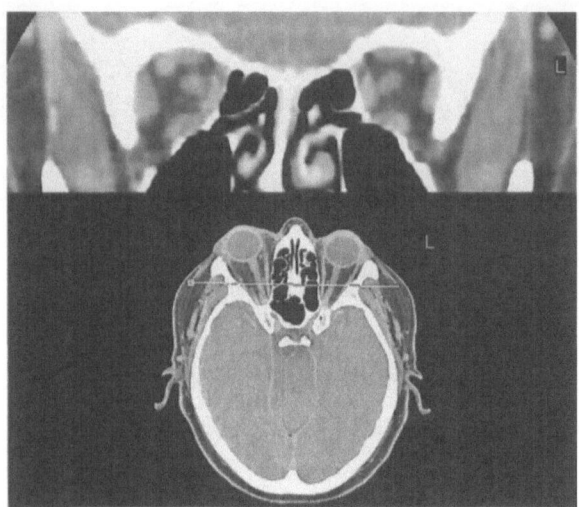

17.5

CT

Enlargement of the right cavernous sinus. Considerable dilatation of the superior ophthalmic vein and its branches. The veins surrounding the trochlea are dilated and elongated. Moderate enlargement of extraocular muscles. Protrusion of the globe.

Diagnosis

Cavernous sinus fistula.

Comment

The CT finding of the enlarged superior ophthalmic vein is typical of cavernous sinus fistula.

K. S., 72-year-old man

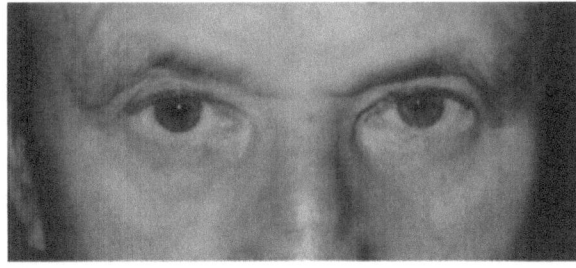

18.1

History and Clinical Findings
Myxoid liposarcomas in the groin, the thoracic wall, and in the adrenal glands, diagnosed 18 months ago.
Complete palsy of the left abducent nerve. Suspicion of a metastasis within the cavernous sinus.

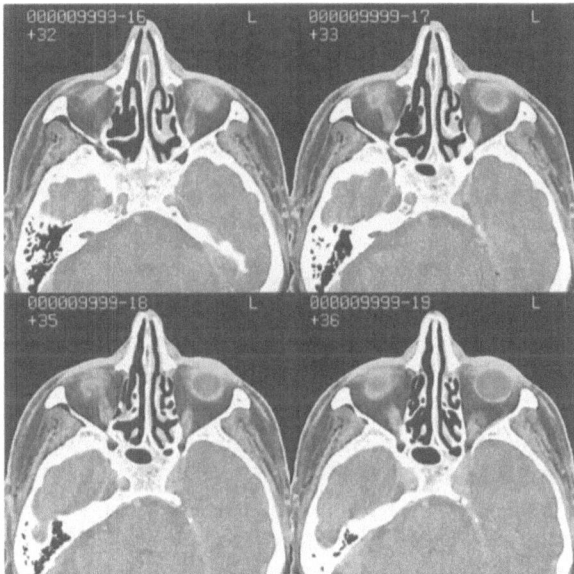

18.2

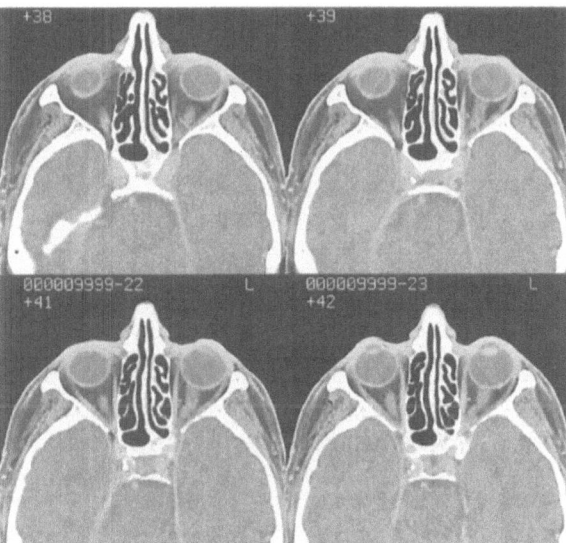

18.3

CT (118.2, 118.3)
The lateral and anterior part of the wall of the left cavernous sinus is convex. The ganglion of the trigeminal nerve is displaced dorsally.

Diagnosis
Slight enlargement of the left cavernous sinus.

Two weeks later, pain "behind the left eye", ptosis, and narrowing of the palpebral fissure (118.6).

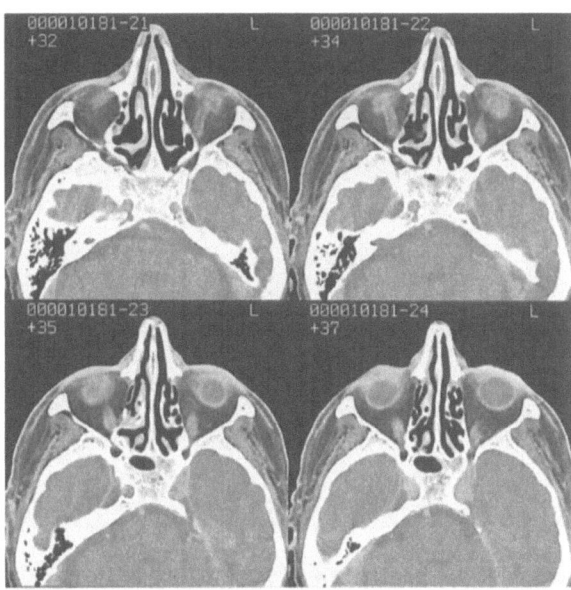

118.4

118.5

CT (118.4, 118.5)
One month later: Increase in the enlargement of the left cavernous sinus. Soft-tissue area within the adjacent superior and anterior part of the left sphenoid bone.

(Continued on p. 168)

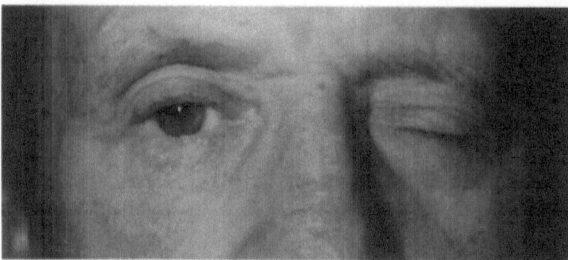

18.6

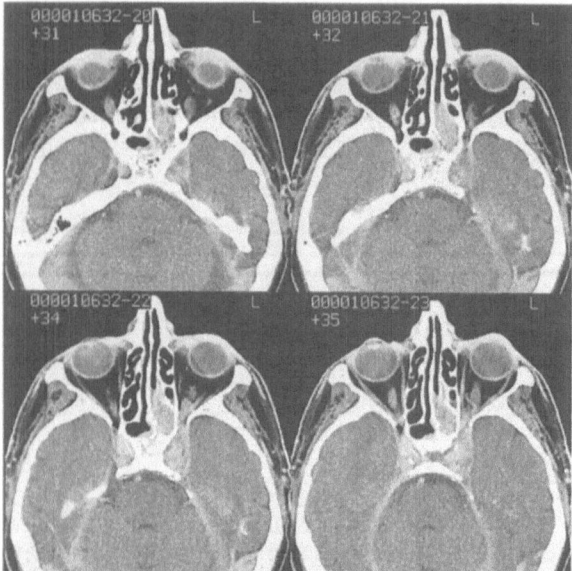

18.7

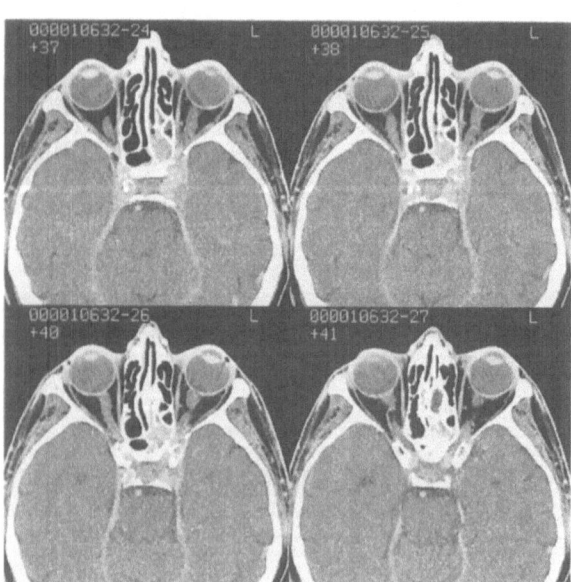

18.8

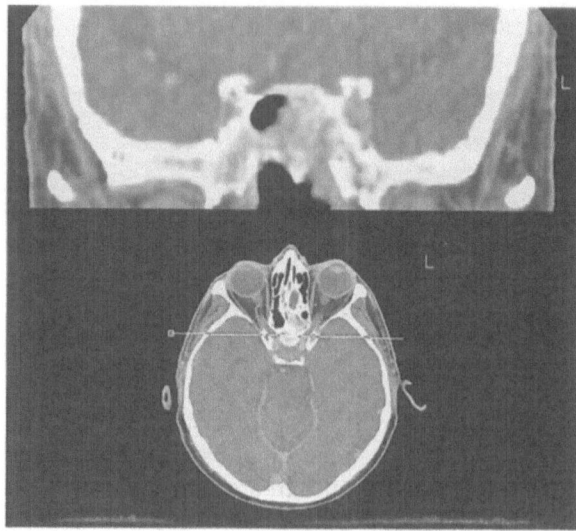

118.9

CT (118.7–118.9)
Three and a half months later: Soft-tissue areas within the dorsal parts of the ethmoidal air cells, the superior and anterior parts of the sphenoid sinuses, the left cavernous sinus, and in the left orbital apex.

Diagnosis
Metastases of the known myxoid liposarcoma (histopathological diagnosis).

Comment
Knowledge of the history of myxoid liposarcoma allowed the diagnosis to be established with a high degree of safety.

Without knowledge of the history, the CT scans could have been misinterpreted as indicative of metastases of other neoplasms, or as a granulo-matous inflammation, such as Wegener's granulo-matosis.

L. F., 66-year-old man

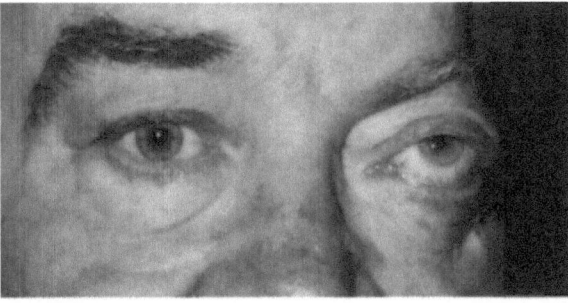

19.1

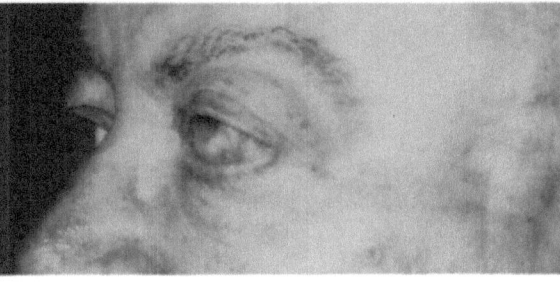

19.2

History and Clinical Findings

Orbitotomies on the left side, performed 16 and 17 years ago. Histopathological diagnosis of the first biopsy was osteoid osteoma. The findings of the second biopsy, were uncertain; a recurrence of the osteoma was assumed.

Radiation therapy.

At present, considerable protrusion of the left globe.

CT

After complete removal of the left lateral orbital wall, the orbital structures are laterally displaced.

Protrusion of the globe. Large, solid calcification above the left medial rectus muscle, which is deformed and enlarged.

Diagnosis

State after lateral orbitotomy on the left side. Deformation and enlargement of the left medial rectus muscle. Large, roundish calcification above the medial rectus muscle.

Clinical Course

The previous surgery and radiotherapy severely obstructed reliable interpretation of CT findings. Therefore, another surgical biopsy was performed.

Histopathology: Liposarcoma.

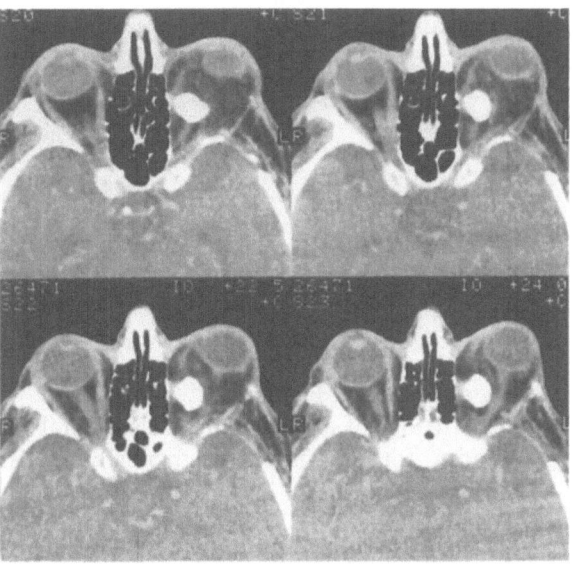

119.3

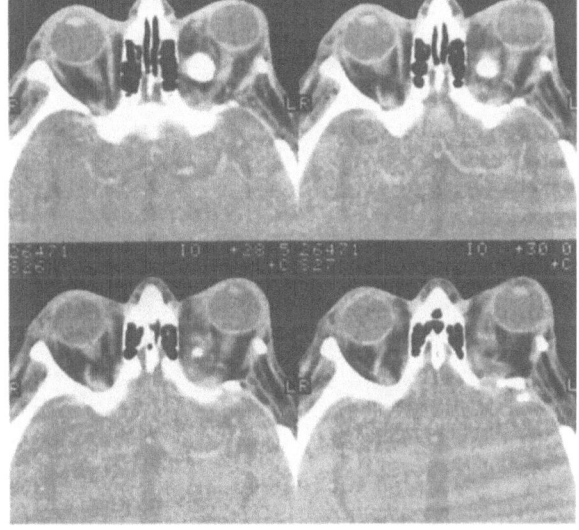

119.4

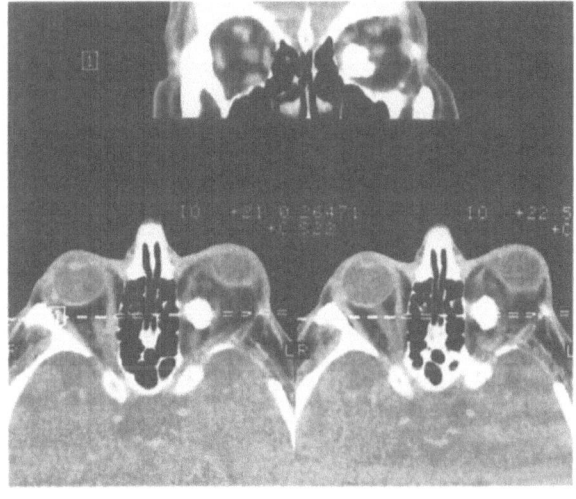

119.5

S. K., 50-year-old woman

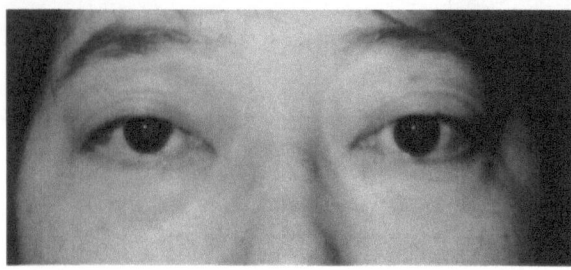

120.1

History and Clinical Findings

A 7-year history of exophthalmos. Near-total thyroidectomy for treatment of hyperthyroidism 3 years ago.

Gradually increasing visual loss in the left eye and intermittent diplopia for the past 18 months.

Presently, the patient is being treated with steroids.

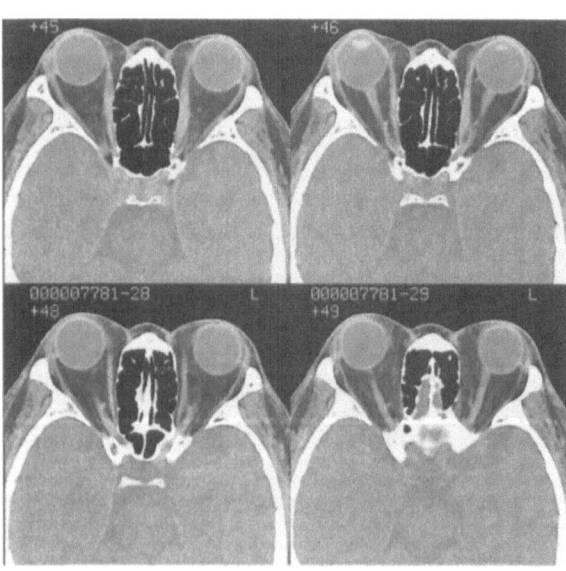

120.2

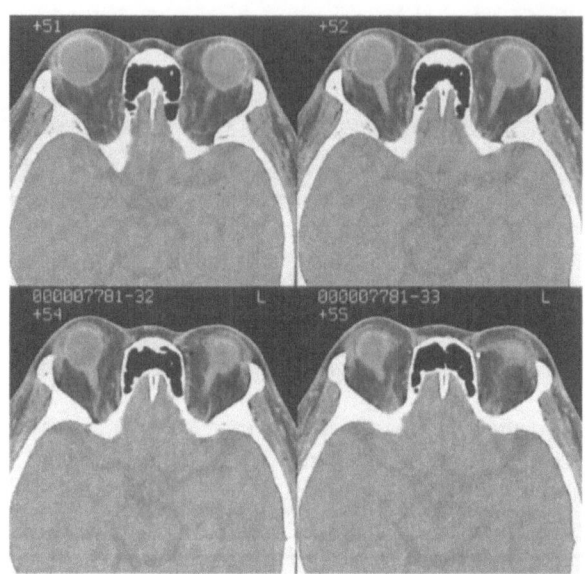

120.3

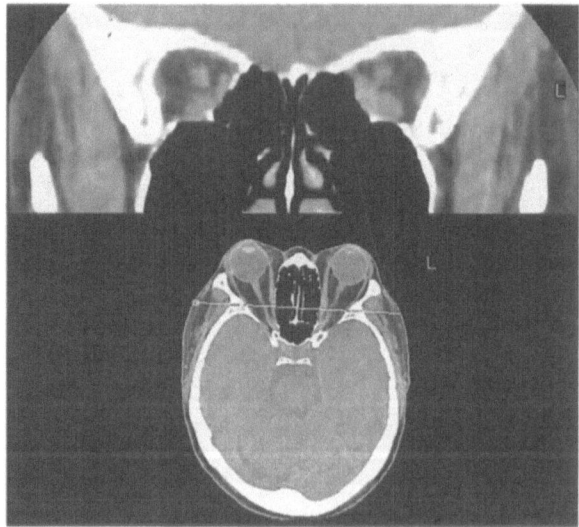

120.4

CT

Slight deformation of both globes consistent with axial myopia. Bilaterally, considerable increase in the volume of the orbital fat. Enlargement of the left medial rectus muscle and of both inferior rectus muscles. Bilateral proptosis.

Diagnosis

Graves' disease. Predominantly, increase in the volume of the orbital fat, combined with moderate enlargement of several extraocular muscles.

Comment

Diplopia is brought about by asymmetrical muscle infiltration.

B. I., 31-year-old woman

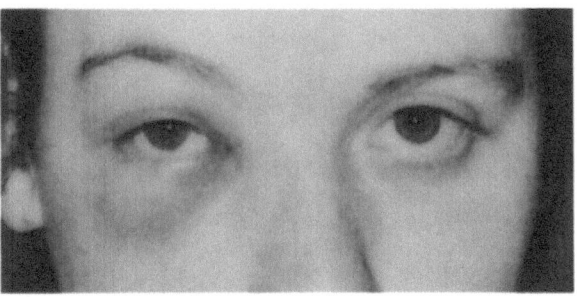

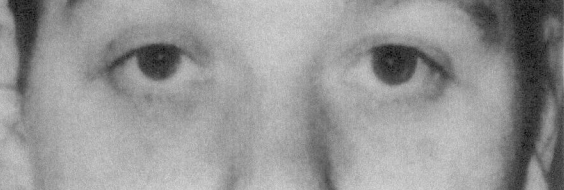

Appearance 3 weeks later (121.3).

History and Clinical Findings
Intermittent itching and a sensation of burning in and around the eyes, as well as chemosis, for the past 5 months.

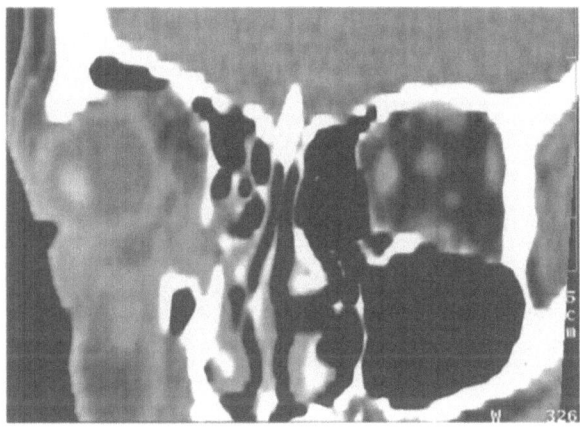

CT (121.2)
Oblique CT reformation showing the right lacrimal sac, the lacrimal duct, and the adjacent nasal cavity: Zones of increased density surrounding the lacrimal sac and extending into the lacrimal duct. Swelling of the mucosa in the adjacent nasal cavity.

Diagnosis
Dacryocystitis.

Clinical Course
Endonasal drainage of purulent matter and lavage. Systemic antibiotic therapy.
    Remission of symptoms within 10 days.

CT image courtesy of the Institute of Radiology and Nuclear Medicine, Grafenberger Allee, Düsseldorf, Germany.

Enlargement of Individual Extraocular Muscles

Plate 15 a

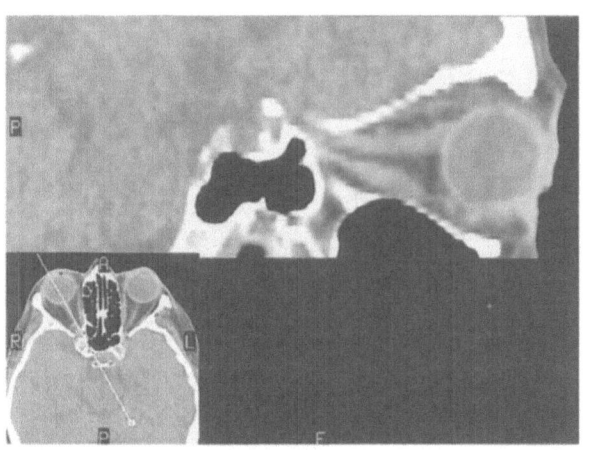

42.1

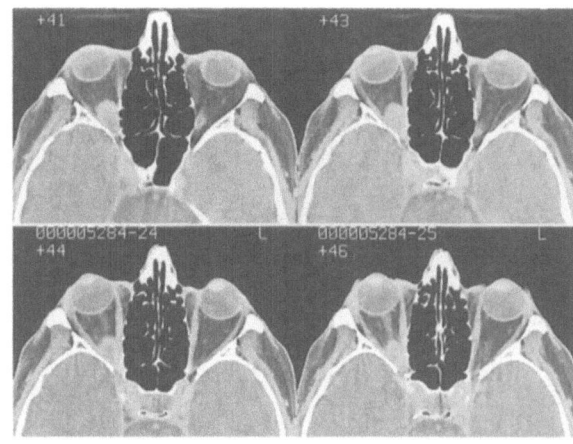

84.1

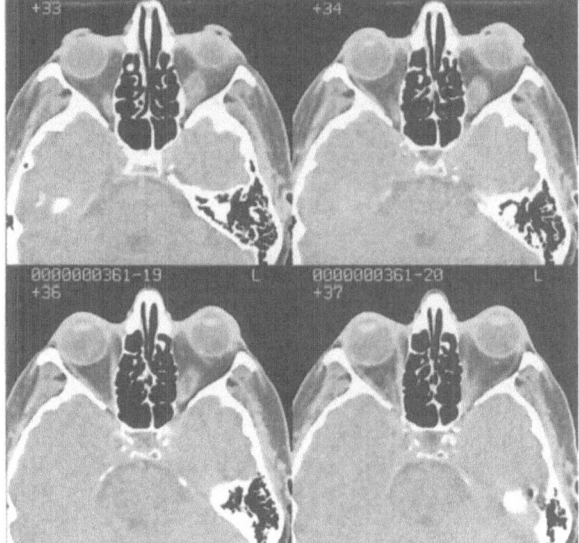

28.2

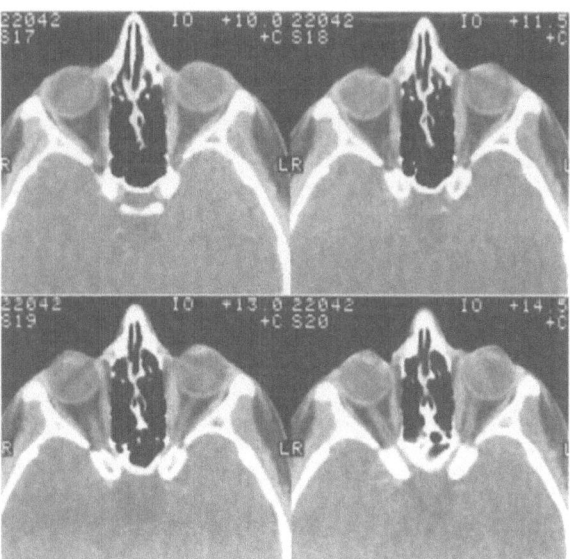

46.1

Case 42.1
Diagnosis: Graves' disease, monomyositic form.

Case 28.2
Diagnosis: Graves' disease, monomyositic form, partial fibrosis of the inferior rectus muscle.

Case 84.1
Diagnosis: Metastasis of a known sqamous cell carcinoma of the lung.

Case 46.1
Diagnosis: Inflammatory orbital pseudotumor, myositic-tendonitic form (left medial rectus muscle).

Enlargement of Individual Extraocular Muscles

Plate 15b

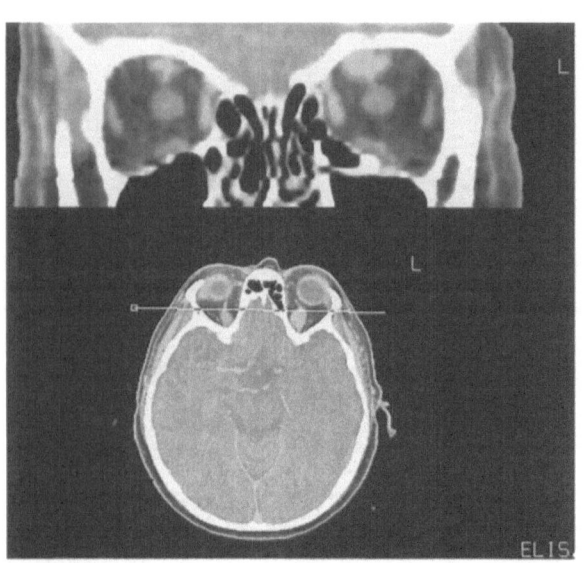

116.5

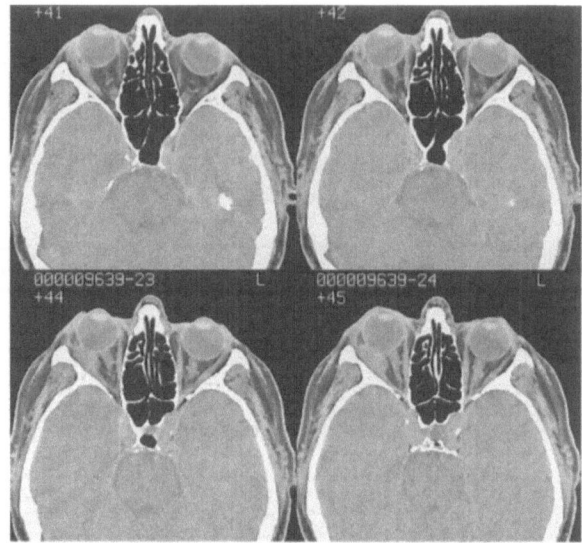

93.1

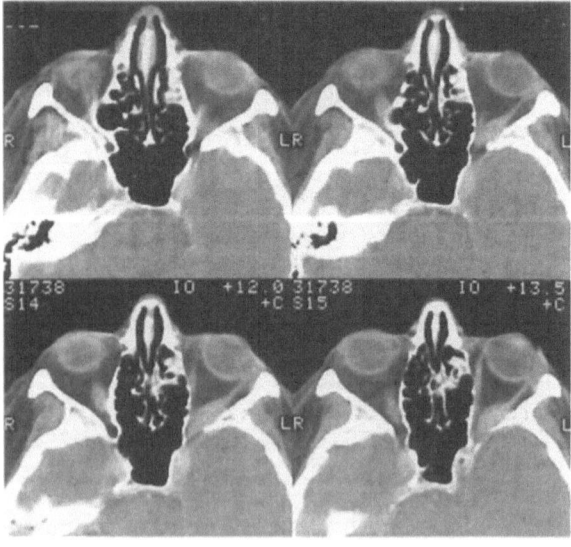

78.1

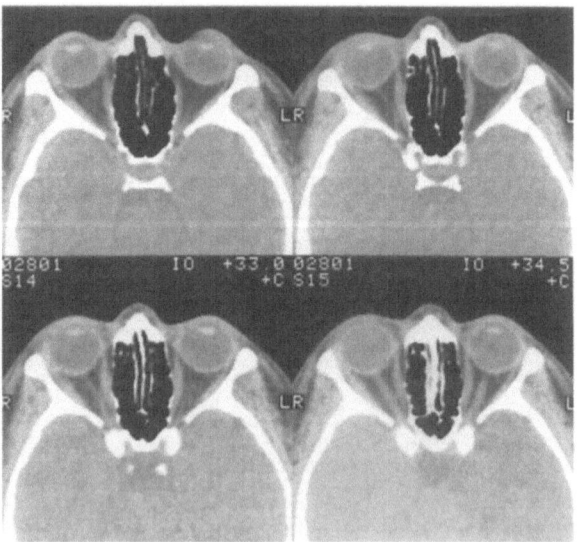

47.1

Case 116.5
Diagnosis: Graves' disease, polymyositic form.

Case 78.1
Diagnosis: Metastasis of an anaplastic carcinoma of the urinary bladder or the cervix.

Case 93.1
Diagnosis: Solitary fibroma in the lateral rectus muscle.

Case 47.1
Diagnosis: Inflammatory orbital pseudotumor, myositic-tendonitic form (right lateral rectus muscle).

Enlargement of Individual Extraocular Muscles

Plate 15 c

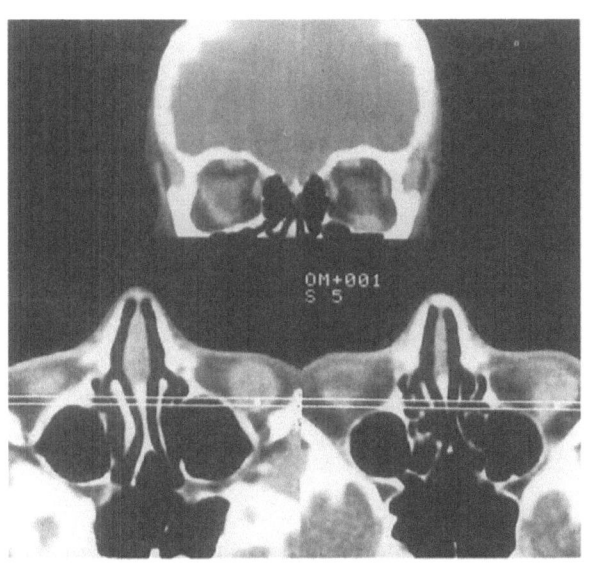

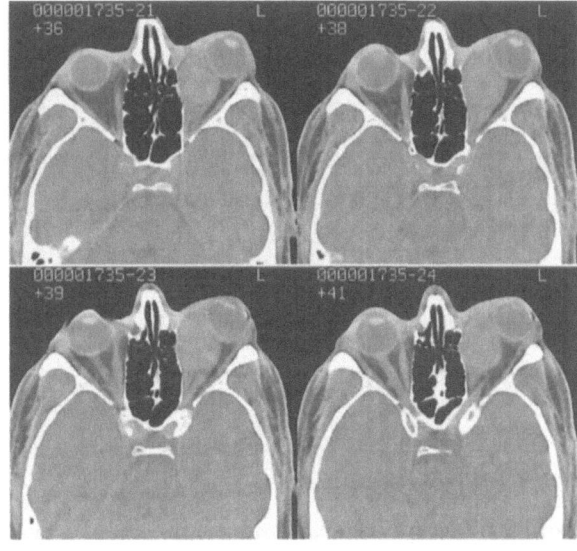

22.1

103.2

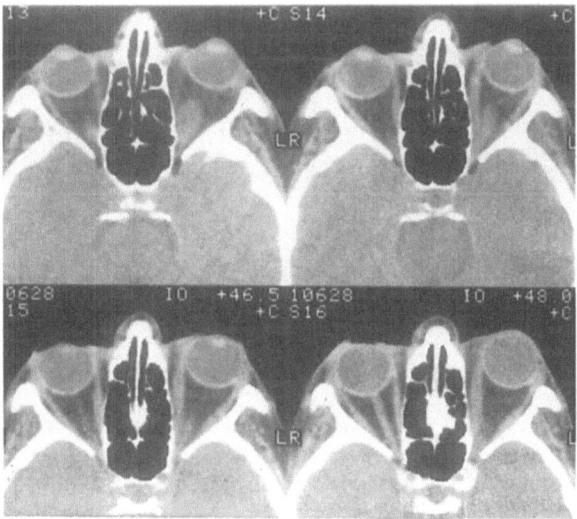

3.1

124.1

Case 122.1
Diagnosis: Granular cell myoblastoma (left inferior oblique muscle).

Case 123.1
Diagnosis: Graves' disease, paucimyositic form (left inferior and medial rectus muscles).

Case 103.2
Diagnosis: Rhabdomyosarcoma (originating in the left medial rectus muscle).

Case 124.1
Diagnosis: Paraneoplastic syndrome in a patient with known gastric carcinoma (no neoplastic infiltration, tendons are involved).

Histopathology of Case 122 courtesy of Professor Heinrich Witschel, Chief of Department of Ophthalmology, Albrecht Ludwigs-University Freiburg, Germany.

Enlargement of Individual Extraocular Muscles

Plate 15 d

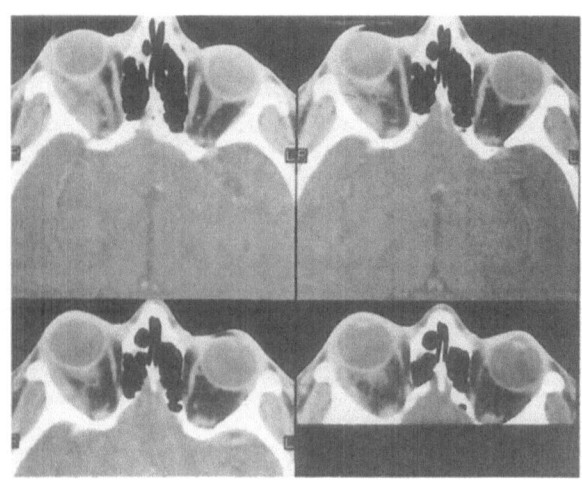

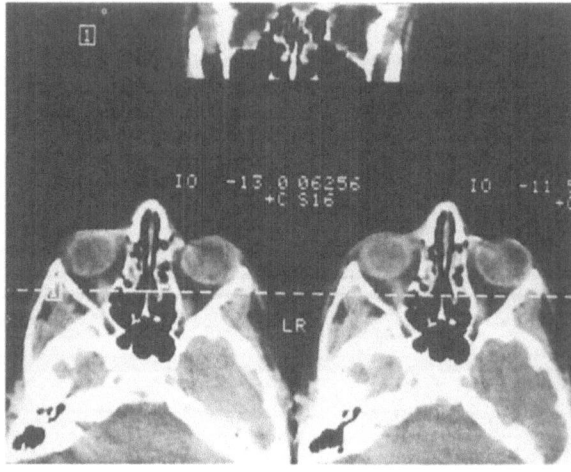

125.1   126.1

Case 125.1
Diagnosis: Myxoid liposarcoma (right lateral rectus muscle).

Case 126.1
Diagnosis: Hematoma within the left inferior rectus muscle.

Diffuse Orbital Infiltration

Plate 16 a

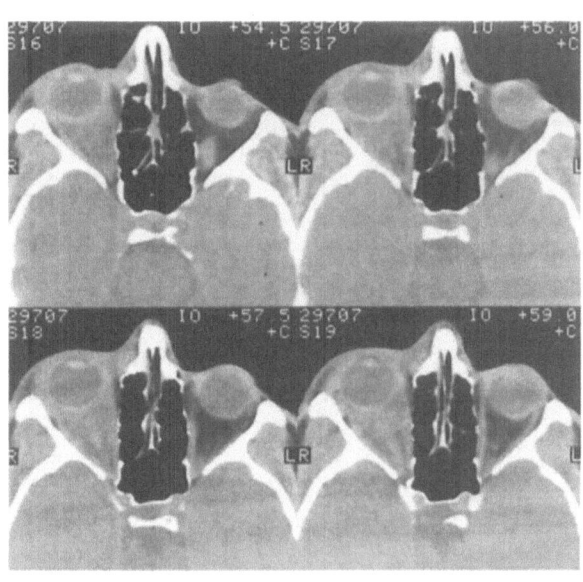

16.2

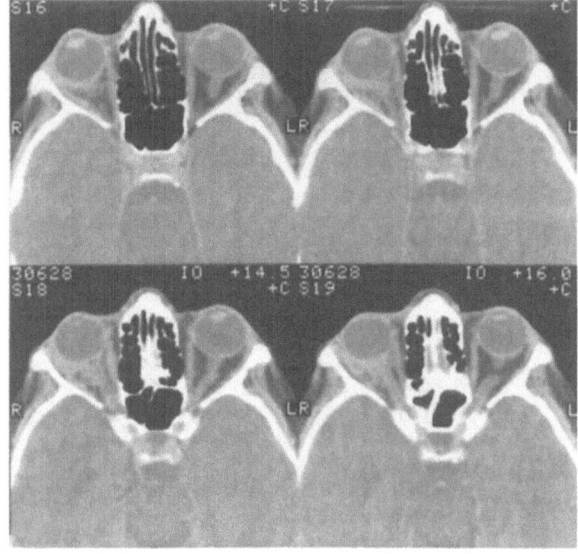

79.2

13.2

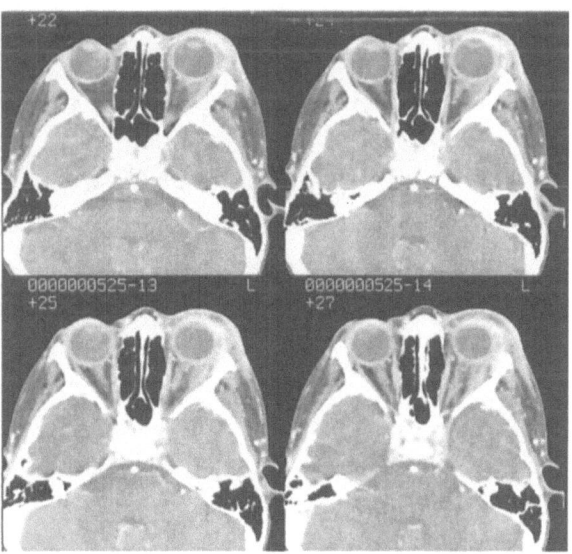

85.2

Case 16.2
Diagnosis: Inflammatory orbital pseudotumor (massive diffusely infiltrating form).

Case 13.2
Diagnosis: Inflammatory orbital pseudotumor (moderate diffusely infiltrating form).

Case 79.2
Diagnosis: Metastasis of a scirrhous carcinoma of the breast.

Case 85.2
Diagnosis: Orbital celllulitis.

Diffuse Orbital Infiltration

Plate 16 b

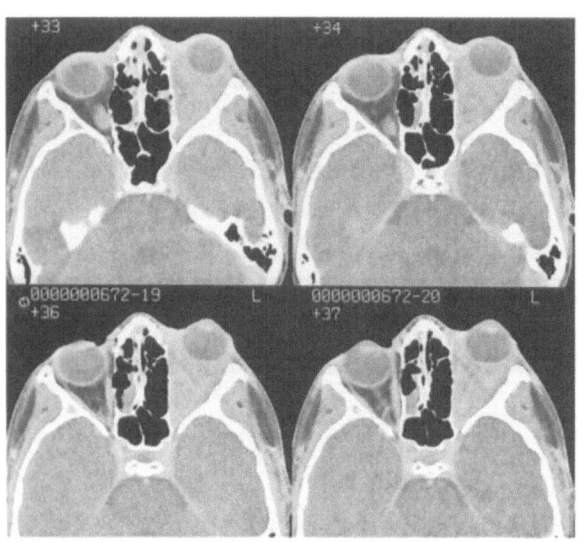

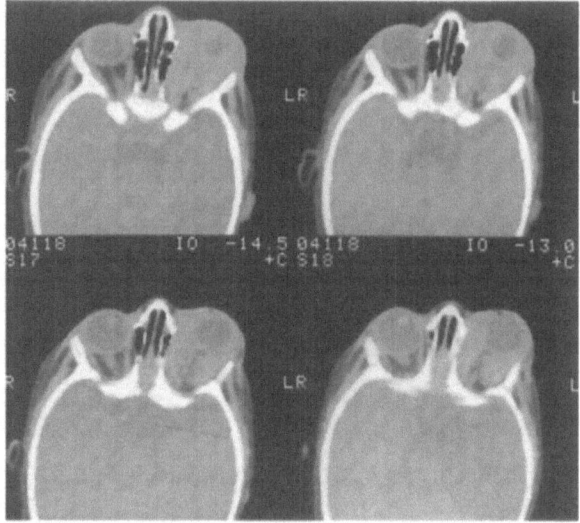

57.3

95.3

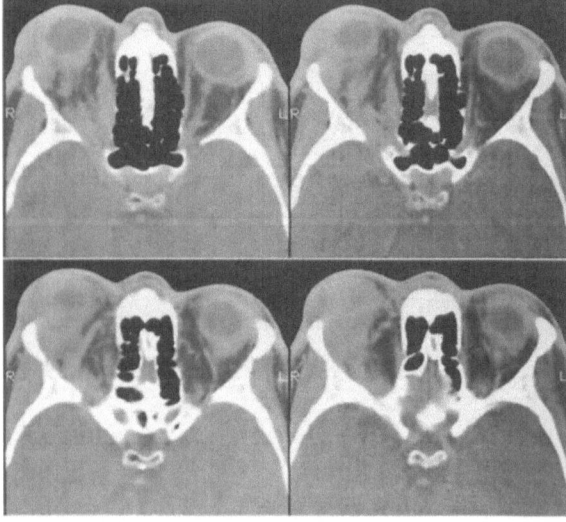

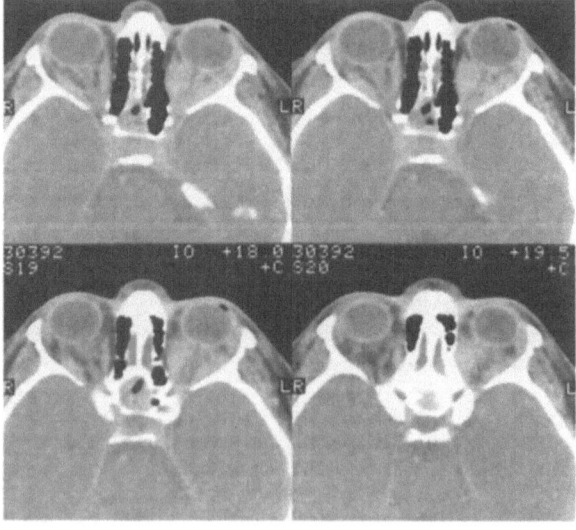

108.2

96.3

Case 57.3
Diagnosis: Inflammatory orbital pseudotumor (massive diffusely infiltrating form).

Case 108.2
Diagnosis: Benign lymphatic hyperplasia consistent with inflammatory orbital pseudotumor.

Case 95.3
Diagnosis: Capillary hemangioma.

Case 96.3
Diagnosis: Metastasis of a scirrhous carcinoma of the breast.

Diffuse Orbital Infiltration

Plate 16c

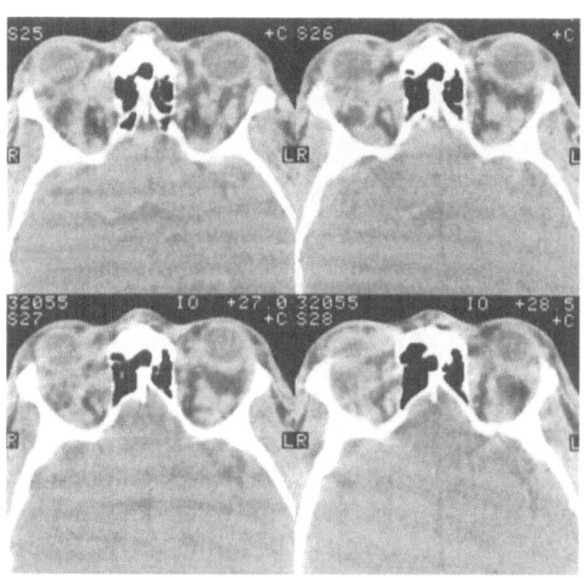

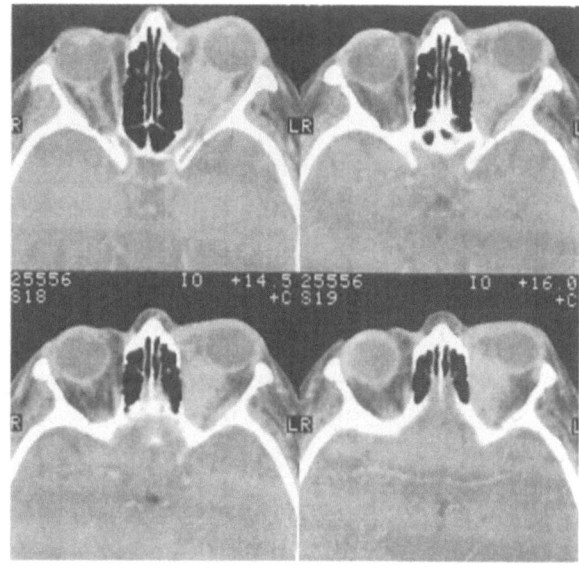

05.4

100.4

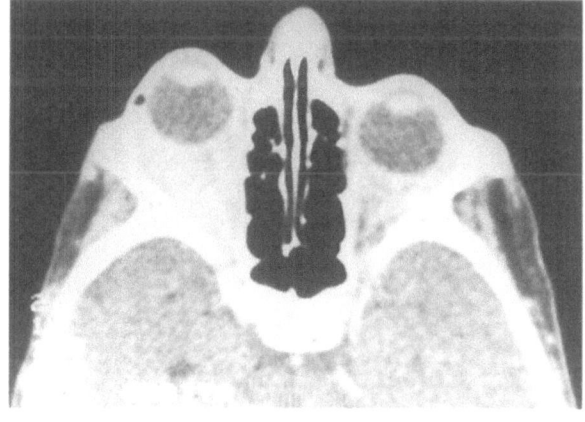

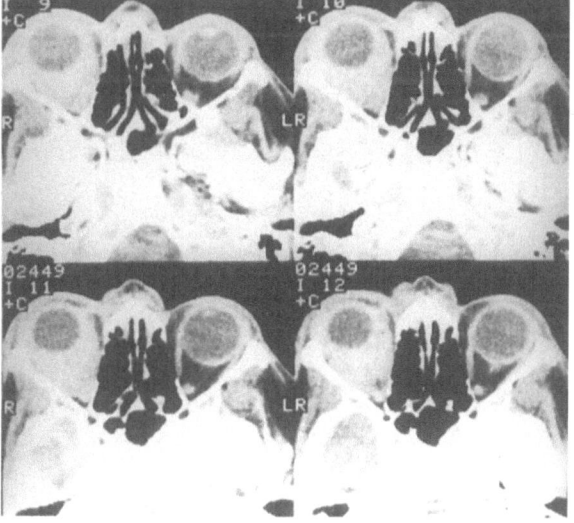

27.1

128.1

Case 105.4
Diagnosis: Non-Hodgkin lymphoma.

Case 100.4
Diagnosis: Metastasis of a carcinoma of the breast.

Case 127.1
Diagnosis: Bilateral inflammatory orbital pseudotumor (massive diffusely infiltrating form).

Case 128.1
Diagnosis: Unilateral inflammatory orbital pseudotumor (massive diffusely infiltrating form).

Diffuse Orbital Infiltration

Plate 16 d

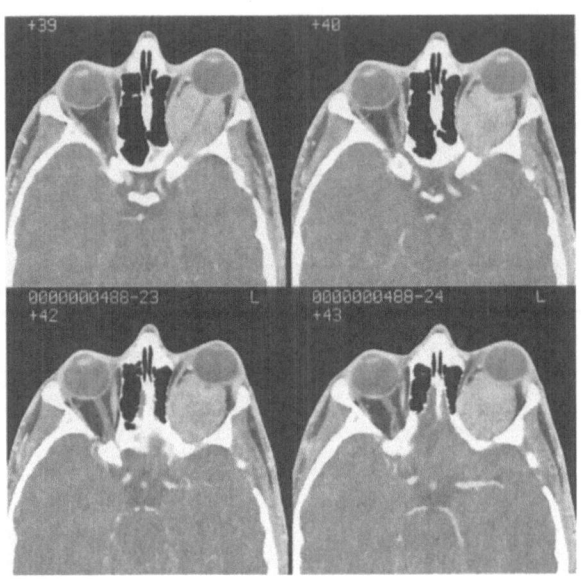

129.1

Case 129.1
Diagnosis: Meningioma of the optic nerve sheath.

Unilateral Enlargement of the Cavernous Sinus

Plate 17 a

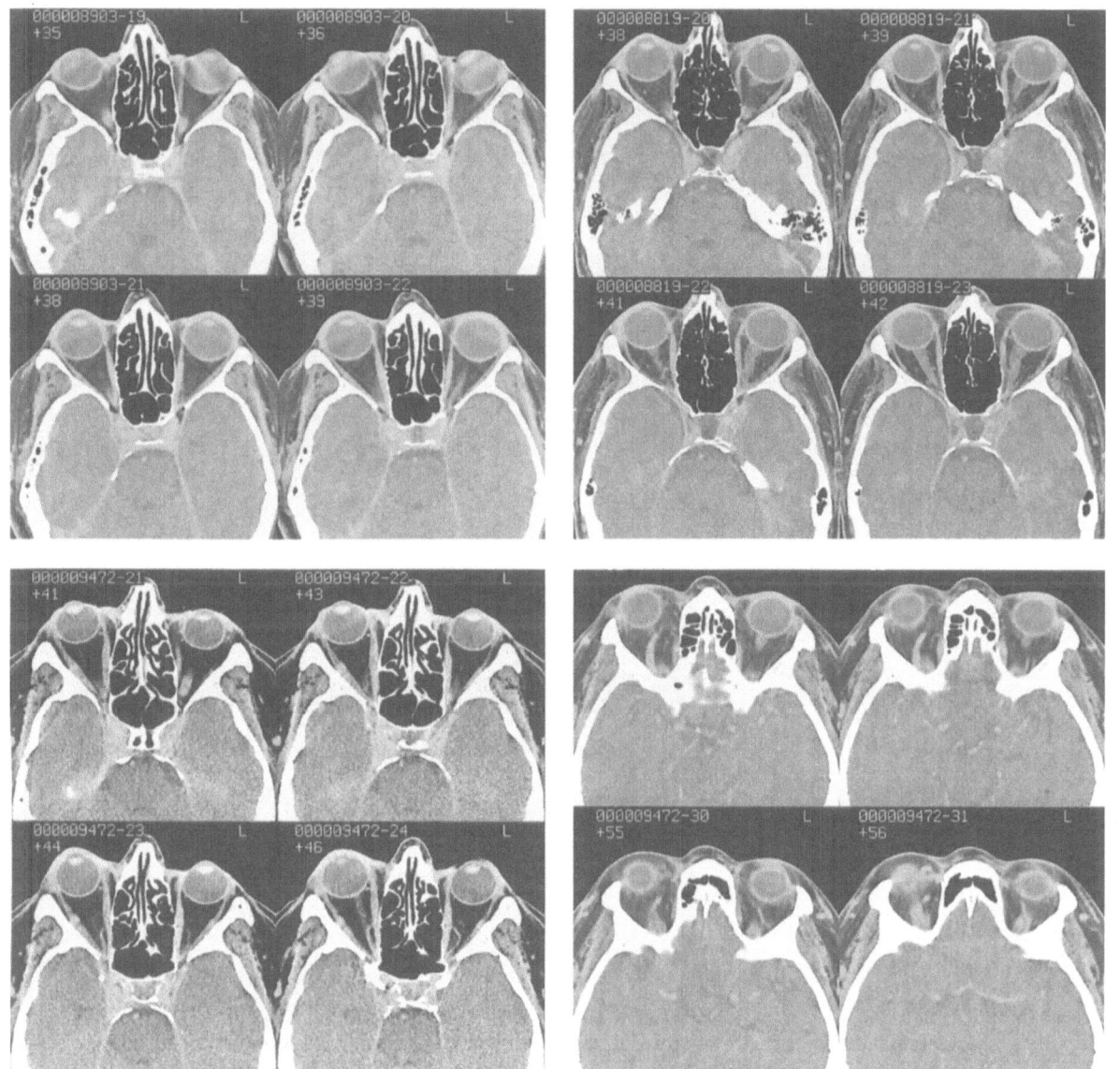

1.1

87.2

7.1

117.2

Case 91.1
Diagnosis: Aneurysm of the right internal carotid artery within the cavernous sinus.

Case 117.1, 2
Diagnosis: Cavernous sinus fistula with dilatation of the right superior ophthalmic vein.

Case 87.2
Diagnosis: Malignant lymphoma infiltrating the left cavernous sinus.

Unilateral Enlargement of the Cavernous Sinus

Plate 17 b

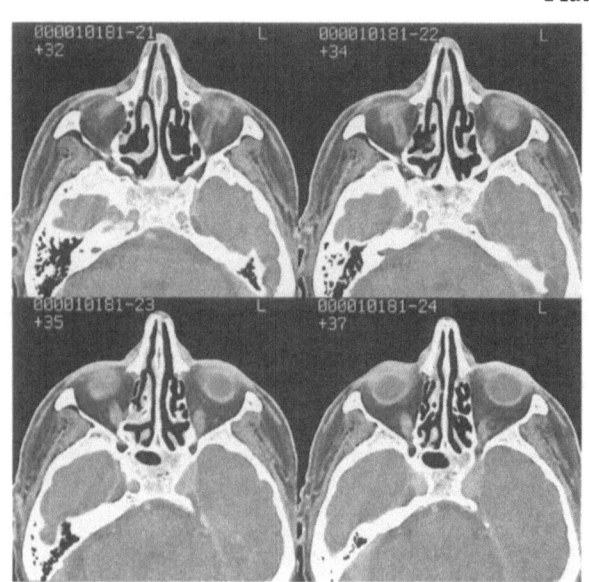

118.5

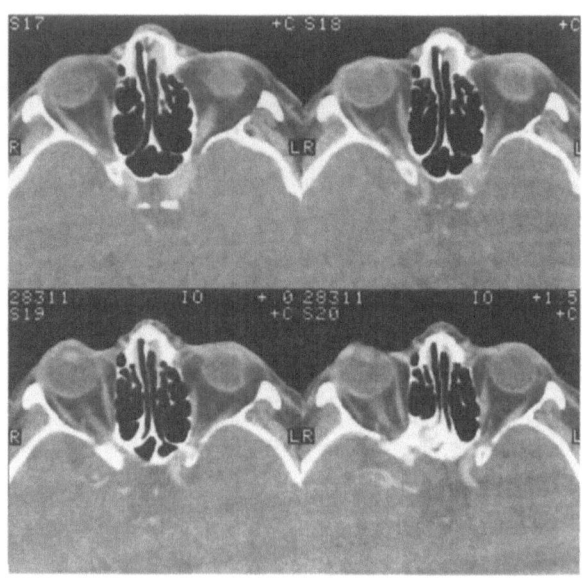

130.1

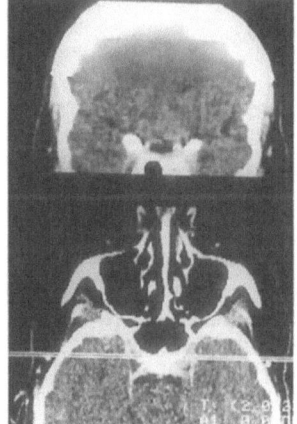

59.2

Case 118.5
Diagnosis: Metastasis of a known myxoid lipo-sarcoma within the left cavernous sinus.

Case 59.2
Diagnosis: Tolosa-Hunt syndrome (Note dilatation of the left cavernous sinus).

Case 130.1
Diagnosis: Dolichoectasia of the internal carotid artery within the left cavernous sinus. (Note additional ectasia of the supraclinoid portion of the left internal carotid artery.)

Plate 18 a

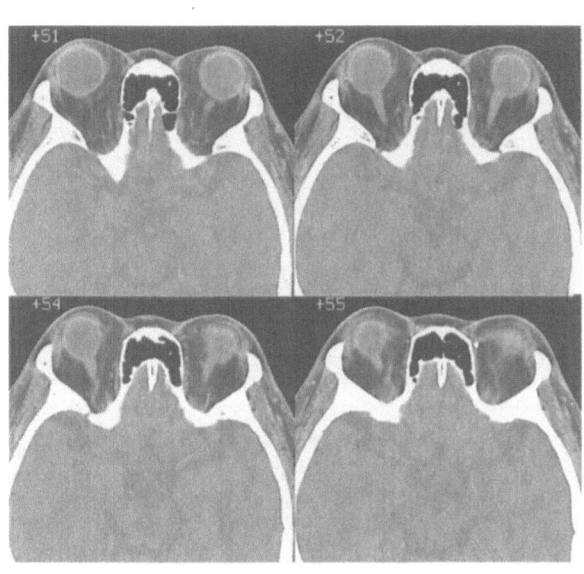

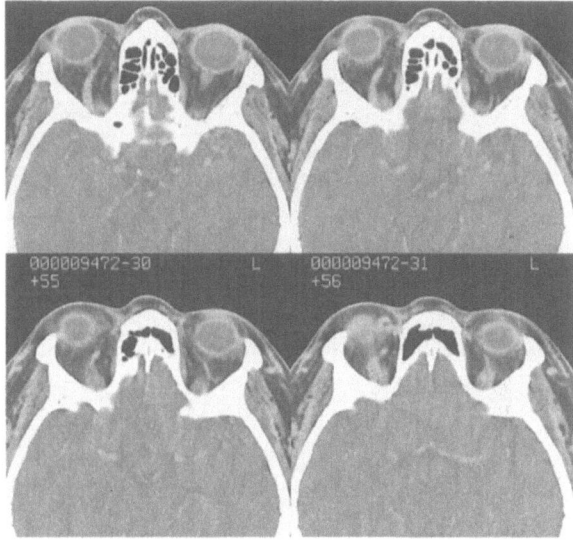

20.3

117.2

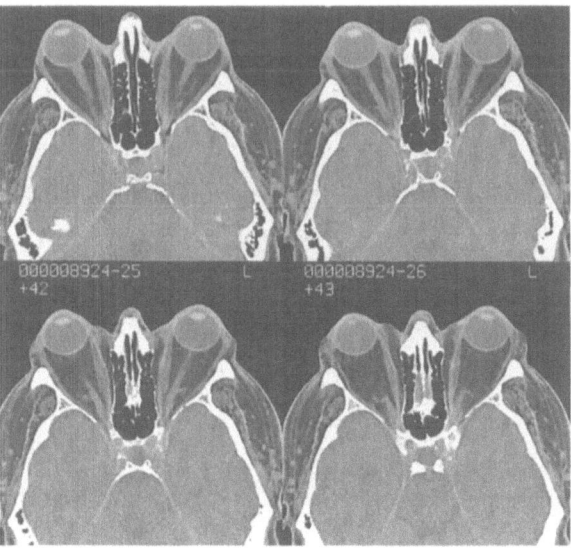

9.3

83.1

Case 120.3
Diagnosis: Graves' disease, predominantly increase in the volume of the orbital fat.

Case 99.3
Diagnosis: Graves' disease, moderate muscle enlargement with secondary fibrosis and increase in the volume of the orbital fat.

Case 117.2
Diagnosis: Cavernous sinus fistula. (Note dilatation of the right superior ophthalmic vein.)

Case 83.1
Diagnosis: Mixed tumor of the lacrimal gland.

Plate 18 b

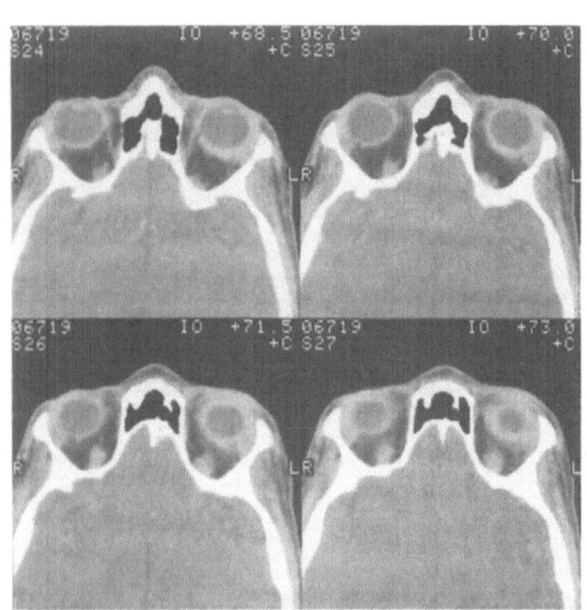

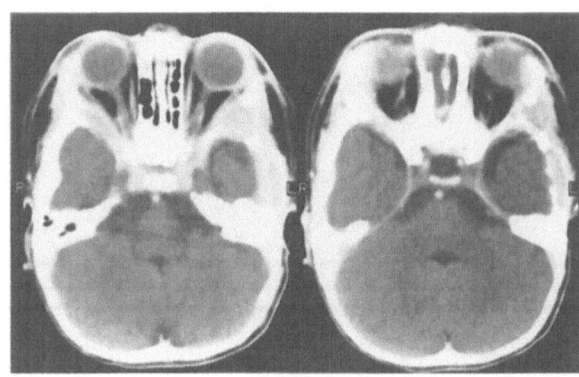

81.3

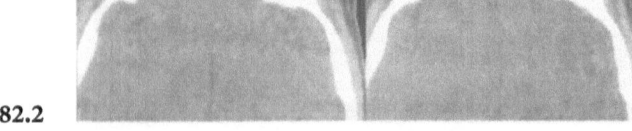

82.2

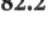

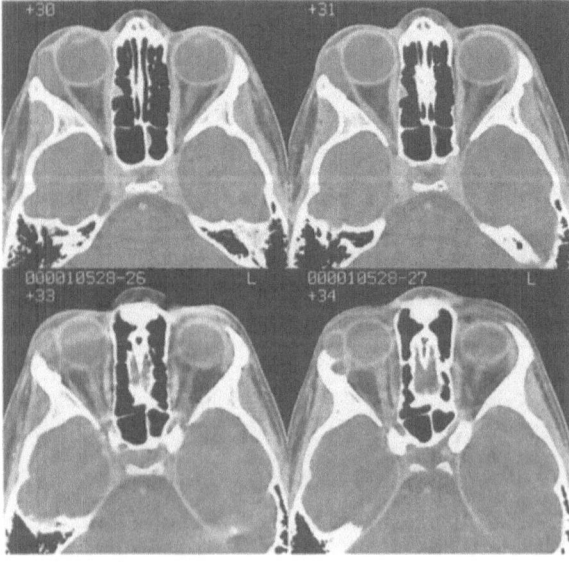

12.3

80.2

Case 82.2
Diagnosis: Inflammatory orbital pseudotumor, scleritic-tenonitic form.

Case 80.2
Diagnosis: Dermoid cyst.

Case 81.3
Diagnosis: Histiocytosis X.

Case 12.3
Diagnosis: Posttraumatic orbital air emphysema.

Plate 18 c

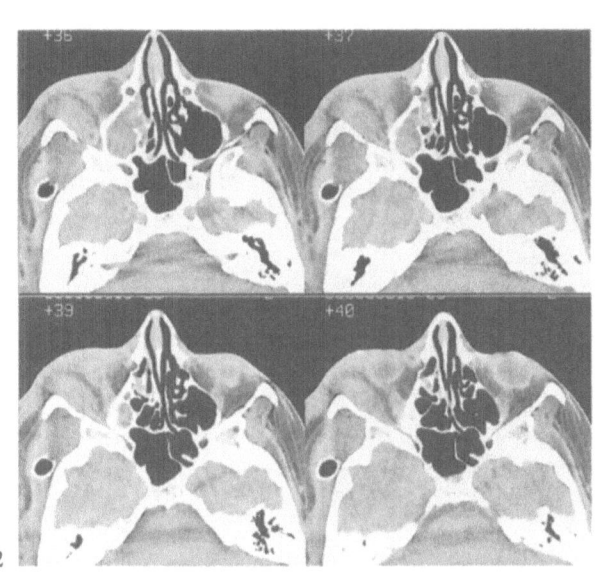

15.2

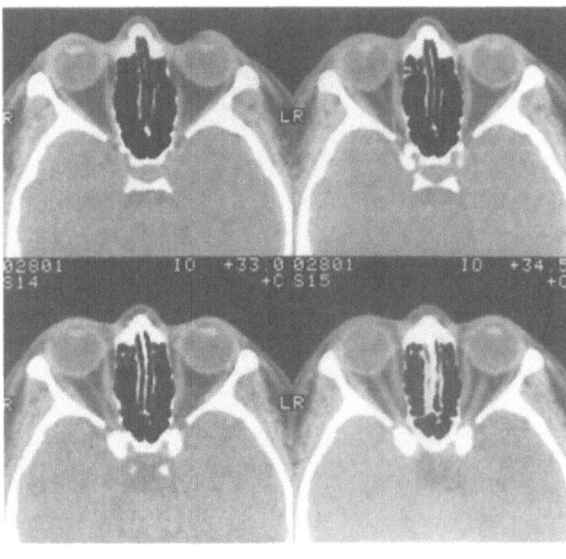

47.1

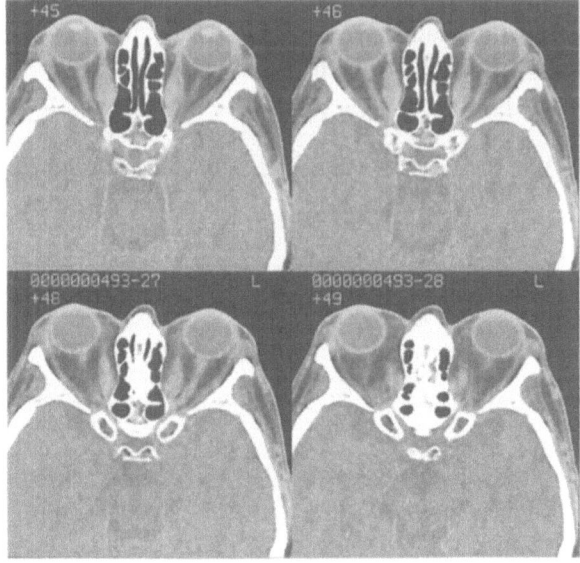

32.2

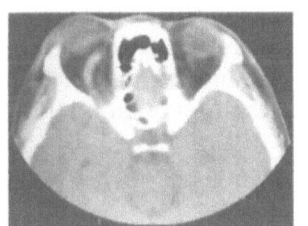

18.2

Case 15.2
Diagnosis: Inflammatory infiltration.

Case 32.2
Diagnosis: Graves' disease.

Case 47.1
Diagnosis: Inflammatory orbital pseudotumor, myositic-tendonitic form (right lateral rectus muscle).

Case 18.2
Diagnosis: Cavernous sinus fistula.

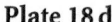

Plate 18 d

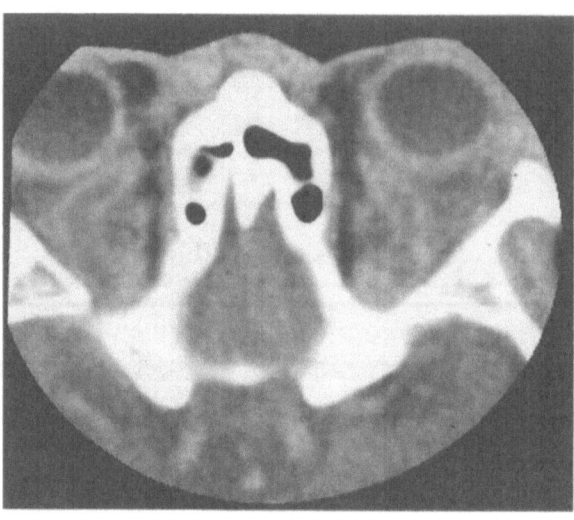

76.2

Case 76.2
Diagnosis: Cavernous sinus thrombosis (Note bilateral dilatation of the superior ophthalmic veins,
the lumina of which appear dark, indicating the
cessation of blood flow).

Bibliography

Antes G (1977) Das primäre gastrointestinale Lymphom. Radiologe 37:35–41

Atlas SW, Bilaniuk LT, Zimmermann RA et al. (1987) Orbit: initial experience with surface coil spin-echo MR imaging at 1.5 T1. Radiology 164:501–509

Bacci V, Giammarco V (1993) "Fiancees" Graves disease. Ann Intern Med 118:232

Bahn RS, Heufelder AE (1992) Retroocular fibroblasts: important effector cells in Graves' ophthalmopathy. Thyroid 2:89–94

Bahn RS, Heufelder AE (1993) Mechanisms of disease: pathogenesis of Graves' ophthalmopathy. N Engl J Med 329:1468–1475

Bartalena L, Marcocci C, Bogazzi F et al. (1989) Use of corticosteroids to prevent progression of Graves' ophthalmopathy after radioiodine therapy for hyperthyroidism. N Engl J Med 321:1349–1352

Becker H, Frisch S (1996) Diagnostische Bedeutung intraorbitaler Verkalkungen im Computertomogramm. Klin Neuroradiol 6:29–35

Birch-Hirschfeld (1905) Zur Diagnostik und Pathologie der Orbitatumoren. Ber Dtsch Ophthalmol Ges 32:127

Blodi FC, Gass JDM (1968) Inflammatory pseudotumour of the orbit. Br J Ophthalmol 52:79

Boergen KP (1991) Ophthalmological diagnosis in autoimmune orbitopathy. Exp Clin Endocrinol 97:235–242

Boergen KP (1993) Augenmuskelveränderungen und ihre Folgen bei endokriner Orbitopathie. Z Prakt Augenheilkd 14:351–356

Boergen KP, Pickardt CR (1991) Neueinteilung der endokrinen Orbitopathien. Med Welt 42:72–76

Borgmann H (1983) „Tolosa-Hunt-Syndrom" – zweijährige Verlaufsbeobachtung. Fortschr Ophthalmol 80: 56–57

Brismar J, Davis KR, Dallow RL, Brismar G (1976) Unilateral endocrine exophthalmos. Diagnostic problems in association with computed tomography. Neuroradiology 12:21–42

Burch HB, Wartofski L (1995) Graves' ophthalmopathy: current concepts regarding pathogenesis and management. Endocr Rev 14:747–793

Char DH, Unsöld R (1990) Computed tomography: ocular and orbital pathology. Clinical aspects. In: Newton TH, Bilaniuk LT (eds) Modern neuroradiology, vol 4: Radiology of the eye and orbit. Raven Press, New York, pp 9.1–9.64

Chung JW, Chang KH, Han MH et al. (1988) Computed tomography of cavernous sinus diseases. Neuroradiology 30:319–328

Dal Pozzo G, Boschi MC (1982) Extraocular muscle enlargement in acromegaly. J Comput Assist Tomogr 6:706–707

Drevelangas A, Kalaitzoglou I, Tsolaki M (1993) Tolosa-Hunt syndrome with sellar erosion: case report. Neuroradiology 35:451–453

Font RL, Gamel JW (1978) Epithelial tumors of the lacrimal gland: an analysis of 265 cases. In: Jakobiec FA (ed) Ocular and adnexal tumors. Aesculapius, Birmingham, Ala, pp 787–805

Forbes GS, Earnest IV F, Waller RR (1982) Computed tomography of orbital tumors, including late-generation scanning techniques. Radiology 142:387–394

Freyschmidt J, Ostertag H (1988) Knochentumoren. Springer, Berlin Heidelberg New York

Frueh BR (1992) Why the NOSPECS classification of Graves' eye disease should be abandoned, with suggestions for the characterization of this disease. Thyroid 2(1):85–88

Gilsbach JM, Unsöld R, Kommerell G et al. (1988) Extended pterional decompression of the orbit: an alternative treatment in endocrine orbitopathy. Neurosurg Rev 11:167–170

Greeven G, Unsöld R (1994) Anleitung zur computertomographischen Untersuchung der Orbita. Schnetztor, Konstanz (conscientia diagnostica)

Hagemann J, Hagemann JR, Arnold H (1983) Varicosis der Orbita im CT. Fortschr Röntgenstr 139:91–93

Handler LC, Davey IC, Hill JC et al. (1991) The acute orbit: differentiation of orbital cellulitis from subperiosteal abscess by computerized tomography. Neuroradiology 33:15–18

Harr DL, Quencer RM, Abrams GW (1982) Computed tomography and ultrasound in the evaluation of orbital infection and pseudotumor. Radiology 142:395–401

Harris GJ (1983) Subperiosteal abscess of the orbit. Arch Ophthalmol 101:751–757

Hasso AN, Pop PM, Thompson JR et al. (1982) High resolution thin section computed tomography of the cavernous sinus. Radiographics 2:83–100

Helmberger T, Schmitt R, Wuttke V (1989) CT-Diagnose einer diffusen Episkleritis. Fortschr Röntgenstr 151: 752–753

Herrmann S, Bachmann G, Zekorn T (1994) Diagnostik der endokrinen Orbitopathie in der Kernspintomographie. Proceedings of the Deutscher Röntgenkongress, Wiesbaden, Germany, 11–14 May 1994

Heufelder AE (1995a) Pathogenesis of Graves' ophthalmopathy: recent controversies and progress. Eur J Endocrinol 132:532–541

Heufelder AE (1995b) Involvement of the fibroblast and TSH receptor in the pathogenesis of Graves' ophthalmopathy. Thyroid 5:331–340

Heufelder AE, Dutton CM, Sarkar G et al. (1993) Detection of TSH receptor RNA in cultured fibroblasts from patients with Graves' ophthalmopathy and pretibial dermopathy. Thyroid 3:297–300

Heufelder AE, Schworm HD, Hofbauer LC (1996) Die endokrine Orbitopathie. Aktueller Stand zur Pathogenese, Diagnostik und Therapie. Dtsch Ärztebl 93:B1043

Hesselink JR, Davis KR, Weber AL et al. (1980) Radiological evaluation of orbital metastases, with emphasis on computed tomography. Radiology 137:363–366

Hirsch M, Lifshitz T (1988) Computerized tomography in the diagnosis and treatment of orbital cellulitis. Pediatr Radiol 18:302–305

Hornblass A, Herschorn BJ, Stern K et al. (1984) Orbital abscess. Surv Ophthalmol 29:169–178

Hosten N, Schörner W, Zwicker C et al. (1991) Lymphozytäre Infiltration der Orbita in MRT and CT. Fortschr Röntgenstr 155:445–451

Hosten N, Lietz A, Noske W, Bechrakis NE (1993) Endokrine Orbitopathie. Korrelation magnetresonanztomographischer und histopathologischer Befunde. Fortschr Röntgenstr 159:304–306

Jakobiec FA, Jones IS (1978) Orbital Inflammations. In: Duane TD (ed) Clinical ophthalmology, vol 2. Harper & Row, Hagerstown, Md, Chap 35:1–75

Joint Committee of European, Japanese, Asia-Oceanian et al. (1992) Classification of eye changes of Graves' disease. Thyroid 2:235–236

Just M, Kahaly G, Higer HP et al. (1991) Graves' ophthalmopathy: role of MR imaging in radiation therapy. Radiology 179:187

Kolokythas O, Brede P, Merkle E (1996) Retrobulbäres pleomorphes Adenom. Röntgenpraxis 49:92–93

Krohel GB, Krauss HR, Winnick J (1982) Orbital abscess. Ophthalmology 89:492–498

Laborde G, Unsöld R, Strunk B et al. (1993) La décompression de l'orbite par voie ptérionale dans le orbitopathies dysthyroidiennes. Neurochirurgie 39:360–368

Lallemand DP, Brasch RC, Char DH et al. (1984) Orbital tumors in children. Radiology 151:85–88

Langer M, Zwicker C, Grannemann D (1987) Kernspintomographische Untersuchungen von orbitalen Raumforderungen. Digit Bilddiagn 7:112–118

Le Hir P, Marsot-Dupuch K, Bigel P et al. (1996) Rhinoscleroma with orbital extension: CT and MRI. Neuroradiology 38:175–178

Lemke A-J, Hosten N, Neumann K et al. (1995) Raumforderungen der Tränendrüse in CT und MRT am Beispiel von vier Fällen. Aktuelle Radiol 5:363–366

Leuenberger S, Signer E (1986) Histiozytose X bei einem 3½jährigen Mädchen mit unklarem Orbitatumor. Klin Monatsbl Augenheilkd 188:486–487

Mackensen G, Unsöld R (1986) Akuter Kopfschmerz aus ophthalmologischer Sicht. In: Lund O-E, Waubke TN (Hrsg) Akute Augenerkrankungen, akute Symptome. Hauptreferate 21. Essener Fortbildung für Augenärzte. Enke, Stuttgart, S 63–75

Mann K (1993) Neues zur Pathogenese des Morbus Basedow. Zusammenfassung und Aspekte für die zukünftige Therapie. In: Reinwein D, Weinheimer B (Hrsg) Schilddrüse 1993. Therapie der Hyperthyreose. 11. Konferenz über die menschliche Schilddrüse, Heidelberg, Henning Symposium. De Gruyter, Berlin, pp 54–59

Mann K (1995) Pathophysiologie des Morbus Basedow und Darstellung häufiger diagnostischer Irrtümer in Morbus Basedow und endokrine Orbitopathie. Häufige Irrtümer bei der Diagnose und typische Fehler bei der Behandlung. In: Pfannenstiel P (ed) Verhandlungsber 13. Wiesbadener Schilddrüsengespräch, Februar 1995

Maroon JC, Kennerdell JS (1976) Lateral microsurgical approach to intraorbital tumors. J Neurosurg 44:556–561

Merlis AL, Schaiberger CL, Adler R (1982) External carotidcavernous sinus fistula simulating unilateral Graves' ophthalmopathy. J Comput Assist Tomogr 6:1006–1009

Mittal BB, Deutsch M, Kennerdell J et al. (1986) Paraocular lymphoid tumors. Radiology 159:793–796

Mödder U, Zanella FE, Lorenz R et al. (1985a) Malignes Lymphom der Orbita, des Gesichtsschädels und des Parapharyngealraumes. Radiologe 25:213–216

Mödder U, Zanella FE, Kirchhof B (1985b) Computertomographie der Orbita. Teil II Iatrogene Veränderungen. Fortschr Röntgenstr 142(6):675–678

Moseley I (1991) Granular cell tumour of the orbit: radiological findings. Neuroradiology 33:399–402

Muhle C, Nölle B, Brinkmann G et al. (1994) Magnetresonanztomographie und Computertomographie der Wegenerschen Granulomatose der Orbita. Aktuelle Radiol 4:229–234

Newton TH, Bilaniuk LT (eds) (1990) Radiology of the eye and orbit, vol IV. Raven Press, New York

Nugent RA, Belkin RI, Neigel JM et al. (1990) Graves orbitopathy: correlation of CT and clinical findings. Radiology 177:675–682

Ohnishi T, Noguchi S, Muramaki N et al. (1993) Levator palpebrae superioris muscle: MR evaluation of enlargement as a cause of upper eyelid retraction in Graves disease. Radiology 188:115–118

Ohnishi T, Noguchi S, Murakami N et al. (1994) Extraocular muscles in Graves ophthalmopathy: usefulness of T2 relaxation time measurements. Radiology 190:857–862

Ostertag CB, Unsöld R, Weigel K (1983) Stereotactic biopsy of orbital lesions. Neuroophthalmology 3(4):277–280

Pappa A, Jackson P, Munro PMG et al. (1993) Glycosaminoglycans in the pathogenesis of thyroid-associated ophthalmopathy. In: Kaufmann H (ed) Transactions 21st Meeting European Strabismological Association, Salzburg, pp 359–363

Peyster RG, Hoover ED (1984) Computerized tomography in orbital disease and neuroophthalmology. Year Book Medical, Chicago

Pickardt CR (1991) Why do we need the ophthalmologist? Exp Clin Endocrinol 97:231–234

Prummel MF, Mourits M, Berghowt A et al. (1991) Prednisone and cyclosporine in the treatment of severe Graves' ophthalmopathy. N Engl J Med 321:1353–1359

Prummel MF, Wiersinga WM (1993) Smoking and risk of Graves' disease. J Am Med Assoc 269:479–482

Rootman J (ed) (1988) Diseases of the orbit. Lippincott, Philadelphia

Rootman J, McCarthy M, White V et al. (1994) Idiopathic sclerosing inflammation of the orbit. A distinct clinico-pathologic entity. Ophthalmology 101:570–584

Rosch PJ (1993) Stressful life events and Graves' disease. Lancet 342:566–567

Rothfus WE, Curtin HD (1984) Extrocular muscle enlargement: a CT review. Radiology 1 51:677–681

Schildwächter A, Unsöld R (1987) Flüchtige Paresen bei Tumoren. Z Prakt Augenheilkd 8:281–285

Schneider G, Tölly E (1984) Radiologische Diagnostik des Gesichtsschädels. Thieme, Stuttgart

Sigmund G, Bähren W, Sigg O et al. (1986) Epidurales Empyem und Orbitaphlegmone. Fortschr Röntgenstr 145:33–37

Sonino N, Girelli ME, Boscaro M et al. (1993) Life events in the pathogenesis of Graves' disease. A controlled study. Acta Endocrinol 128:293–296

Stammen J, Unsöld R, Greeven G (1995) Computertomographische Befunde bei akutem Brown-Syndrom. Sitzungsber 157. Versammlung Rhein.-Westf. Augenärzte, Aachen, pp 139–146

Towbin R, Han BK, Kaufman RA et al. (1986) Postseptal cellulitis: CT in diagnosis and management. Radiology 158:735–737

Trattnig S, Eilenberger M, Schurawitzki H et al. (1991) Varicosis orbitalis. Fortschr Röntgenstr 155:207–210

Trokel SL, Sadek KH (1979) Recognition and differential diagnosis of enlarged extraocular muscles in computed tomography. Am J Ophthalmol 87:503–512

Uhlenbrock D, Becker W, Appel W et al. (1983) Die alte und neu aufgetretene endokrine Ophthalmopathie in der Computertomographie. Gemeinsamkeiten – Unterschiede. Fortschr Röntgenstr 139:644–647

Unsöld R (1982) Zur computertomographischen Differentialdiagnose der Erkrankungen des Sehnerven. Graefes Arch Clin Exp Ophthalmol 218:124–138

Unsöld R (1984a) Differentialdiagnose chronisch-entzündlicher Orbitaprozesse unter Verwendung der Computertomographie. In: Lund O-E, Waubke T (eds) Die chronisch-entzündlichen Erkrankungen des Auges. Hauptreferate 19. Essener Fortbildung für Augenärzte. Enke, Stuttgart, pp 142–155

Unsöld R (1984b) Die Bedeutung der Computer-Tomographie für die Diagnose orbitaler Traumen. Fortschr Ophthalmol 81:579–582

Unsöld R (1985) CT-Orbitadiagnostik im Kindesalter. In: Lund OE, Waubke TN (eds) Die Augenerkrankungen im Kindesalter. Hauptreferate 20. Essener Fortbildung für Augenärzte. Enke, Stuttgart, pp 218–225

Unsöld R (1989) Computertomographische Befunde bei endokriner Orbitopathie. Ihre differentialdiagnostische und therapeutische Bedeutung. Sitzungsber 151. Versammlung Rhein.-Westfäl. Augenärzte, Münster, pp 87–89

Unsöld R (1993) Radiologische Befunde bei Exophthalmus. In: Lund OE, Waubke TN (eds) Neuroophthalmologie. Hauptreferate 28. Essener Fortbildung für Augenärzte. Enke, Stuttgart, pp 146–155

Unsöld R, Seeger W (1989) Compressive optic nerve lesions at the optic canal. Springer, Berlin Heidelberg New York

Unsöld R, Hoyt WF, Newton TH (1979) Die computertomographischen Merkmale des kavernösen Hämangioms und ihre Bedeutung für die Differentialdiagnose im Muskeltrichter gelegener Tumoren der Orbita. Klin Monatsbl Augenheilkd 175:773–785

Unsöld R, Newton TH, DeGroot J (1980a) CT evaluation of extraocular muscles. Anatomic-CT correlations. Graefes Arch Klin Exp Ophthalmol 214:155–180

Unsöld R, Ostertag C, Newton TH (1980b) Zur Differentialdiagnose endokriner Orbitopathien und entzündlicher Pseudotumoren der Orbita. Computertomographie-Befunde. Klin Monatsbl Augenheilkd 177:31–47

Unsöld R, DeGroot J, Newton TH (1980c) Images of the optic nerve: anatomic-CT correlation. Am J Neuroradiol 1:317–323

Unsöld R, Feldon S, Newton TH (1981) Zur Diagnose orbitaler Muskelerkrankungen. Klinische Anwendung von Computer-Rekonstruktionen. Klin Monatsbl Augenheilkd 178:436–438

Unsöld R, Ostertag CB, DeGroot J et al. (1982) Computer reformations of the brain and skull base. Springer, Berlin Heidelberg New York

Vana S, Nemec J, Rezek P et al. (1992) Langfristige Resultate der Therapie bei endokriner Orbitopathie. Totale thyreoidale Ablation in Kombination mit Prednisolon verbessert die Erfolge. In: Röher HD, Weinheimer B (eds) Schilddrüse 1991: Therapie der Struma. 10. Konferenz über die menschliche Schilddrüse, Heidelberg, Henning Symposium. De Gruyter, Berlin, pp 432–439

Vargas ME, Warren FA, Kupersmith MJ (1993) Exotropia as a sign of myasthenia gravis in dysthyroid ophthalmopathy. Br J Ophthalmol 77:822–823

Werner SC (1977) Modification of the classification of the eye changes of Graves' disease. Am J Ophthalmol 83:725–727

Winsa B, Adami H-O, Bergström R et al. (1991) Stressful life events and Graves' disease. Lancet 338:1475–1479

Subject Index